ADVANCE PRAISE FOR

Diabetes: Sugar-Coated Crisis

Eloquent and thought-provoking.
— RICHARD RUBIN, PhD, author of *Psyching Out Diabetes*,
and American Diabetes Association President for
. Health Care and Education

With deep understanding, intelligence and passion,
David Spero shines a bright light on the social and
environmental determinants that underlie diabetes and
other chronic illnesses. David, a highly effective clinician,
peer counselor and coach, also inspires, empowers and
encourages readers to take actions to promote personal well-
being as well as actions that will improve the lives of others.
— MICHAEL G. GOLDSTEIN, MD, Associate Director,
Clinical Education and Research, Institute for
Healthcare Communication

Diabetes: Sugar-Coated Crisis had to be written.
It proves we can transcend the standard medical model
characterized by brilliant science applied without wisdom.
In David Spero's book, human wisdom supports science,
and science serves not only medical but also social truth.
— DR. GABOR MATÉ, from the foreword

David Spero has struck the right note in taking readers
through a tour of how poverty and public policy have
contributed to the deadly epidemic of diabetes.
— DORIANE MILLER MD, National Program Director,
Quality Allies: Improving Care by Engaging Patients, a
program of the Institute for Healthcare Improvement

We read almost daily about the diabetes epidemic, and we know about the ever-increasing rates of obesity. But Spero digs far deeper to see what is behind this epidemic — how our social environment and economic distribution are prominent causes. We need to address these issues at all levels, if we are to improve lives and health. Spero's book clearly and powerfully speaks to how we can do this.

— LAURIE FRANCIS, MPH, Chief Executive Officer, Community Health Partners

A compelling and inspiring resource for people, communities, and health systems struggling with diabetes and other chronic conditions.

— DR. AMERICA BRACHO, MPH, CDE, President and CEO, Latino Health Access

DIABETES:
SUGAR-COATED CRISIS

DIABETES:
SUGAR-COATED CRISIS

WHO GETS IT,
WHO PROFITS AND
HOW TO STOP IT

DAVID SPERO, RN

with a foreword by **GABOR MATÉ**, MD

NEW SOCIETY PUBLISHERS

CATALOGING IN PUBLICATION DATA
A catalog record for this publication is available from the National
Library of Canada.

Cover design by Diane McIntosh. Photo: Alamy/Comstock

Printed in Canada. First printing August 2006.

Paperback ISBN 13: 978-0-86571-567-7
Paperback ISBN 10: 0-86571-567-x

Inquiries regarding requests to reprint all or part of *Diabetes: Sugar-Coated Crisis* should be addressed to New Society Publishers at the address below.

To order directly from the publishers, please call toll-free (North America) 1-800-567-6772, or order online at www.newsociety.com

Any other inquiries can be directed by mail to:

New Society Publishers
P.O. Box 189, Gabriola Island, BC VOR 1X0, Canada
1-800-567-6772

New Society Publishers' mission is to publish books that contribute in fundamental ways to building an ecologically sustainable and just society, and to do so with the least possible impact on the environment, in a manner that models this vision. We are committed to doing this not just through education, but through action. We are acting on our commitment to the world's remaining ancient forests by phasing out our paper supply from ancient forests worldwide. This book is one step toward ending global deforestation and climate change. It is printed on acid-free paper that is 100% old growth forest-free (100% post-consumer recycled), processed chlorine free, and printed with vegetable-based, low-VOC inks. For further information, or to browse our full list of books and purchase securely, visit our website at: www.newsociety.com

NEW SOCIETY PUBLISHERS   www.newsociety.com

To O. Brion Whitford

Contents

Acknowledgments

YOU CAN'T THANK EVERYBODY, but here's a sampling: June Spero, my editor, supporter and mother; Alf Adams, my best critic, editor and comrade. Aisha, Sekani, Mathias (Sarge), Rachel, Daniel, Jonathan, Ira, Donna, Ron, Lauren, Sharon and the younger generation. The New Society team: Chris, Ingrid, Bethanne, Judith and everybody. Albert, Lotus, Bob, Gail, David S., Kim, Ralph, Leslie and all the friends and people who wish me well. Jane, Shirley, Hose, Steve, Karen, Frank, Dolores, Mario, Robin and the rest of the MS group.

The heroes I've met: Cheryl Sampson (Agnaqin), Ane McDonald, Regina Whitewolf, Ann Bullock, Hilary Zepeda, Josephine Malamute, Sarah Vent and other indigenous heart warriors. America Bracho, Caleb Arias, Melanie Tervalon, Kimi Watkins-Tartt, Mark Alexander, Gigi Gregory, Amanda Aguirre, Elaine Peacock and the other community builders.

James Ratliff, Eliot Brown, Marilyn Montoya, Richard Bernstein and the other self-care role models.

Kate Lorig, Athena Philis-Tsimikis, Devin Sawyer, David Sobel, Thomas Bodenheimer and the others who are revolutionizing medicine from within.

Marti Funnell, Carla Gentry, Mary Leighton, Karen Weissman, Ann Williams and all the great diabetes educators.

The psychologists: Bill Polonsky, Richard Rubin, Robert Anderson, Kelly Brownell. The geniuses of social science: Leonard Syme, Nancy Adler, Gabor Maté, Richard Wilkinson, Michael Marmot, Paul Gilbert, Elissa Epel; and of experimental science: Michael Meaney, Patrick Lustman, Albert Bandura, et al. The journalists: Eric Schlosser, Greg Critser and all the reporters who first found these amazing stories.

And to everyone who helped make this book a reality, and everyone who is striving toward wellness for themselves, their communities and the world. If you wonder if you belong on that list, believe me, you do. Thank you for giving me hope.

Foreword

by Dr. Gabor Maté

IN *DIABETES: SUGAR-COATED CRISIS,* David Spero sets himself the task of placing diabetes in context. Rather than seeing this disease, reaching epidemic proportions in North America, as a failure of a particular organ or organs in an isolated human body, he presents it as the consequence of social and economic forces that deprive people of power in their lives. In this endeavor Spero stands on solid ground. Science has proven that a person's physiology cannot be separated from his or her emotions, nor from the emotional, social, economic and political environment in which that person develops, lives and works. Our psychology and physiology are both shaped by the milieu in which we function.

It is no accident, as Spero documents, that minority populations with a history of oppression and who continue to face discrimination are at greater risk for many diseases, including and especially diabetes. Stress, he points out, is not an abstract psychological event but a physical set of responses in the body. The end point is the release of cortisol: the hormone responsible for raising blood sugar. Stressed populations, therefore, are high risk populations for diabetes. And lack of power, the stress literature clearly shows, is a major stressor.

People without a sense of power in their lives are also easier prey for the purveyors of the junk comfort foods that make up so much of the North American diet. Refined sugar, Spero points out, has a direct addictive effect through the release of endorphins, the body's intrinsic opiate compounds. Junk food addiction, to which groups low on the socio-economic scale are more prone, is a socially engineered risk factor for diabetes. In our profit-driven and highly manipulated society, of course, stress and a loss of personal agency are hardly restricted to minority populations. Anyone, regardless of social position, is at risk. Simply put, people emotionally or socially stressed or disempowered are less likely to take good care of themselves.

David Spero does more than document the social dynamics that drive the diabetes epidemic. In well-researched and clearly thought out chapters, he proposes solutions from which both patients and medical caregivers will benefit. The key is to empower the individual by connecting him or her with sources of information and also with other people. The medical model has an unfortunate tendency, often despite even the best intentions of physicians, to deprive patients of power. It does so by making the doctor the repository of knowledge and the dispenser of healing. Spero's intent, in which his book succeeds admirably, is to place the person with diabetes at the centre.

Diabetes, Spero argues, is not an irreversible condition. In many cases, its progress can not only be arrested, but most or all of its physiological and laboratory manifestations can be eliminated. More than that, given social and political will, diabetes could be largely prevented. Whatever genetic predispositions may contribute to it, for the most part these need not be decisive if the environmental conditions that feed it are controlled.

Diabetes: Sugar-Coated Crisis had to be written. It proves we can transcend the standard medical model characterized by brilliant science applied without wisdom. In David Spero's book, human wisdom supports science, and science serves not only medical but also social truth.

— Gabor Maté, MD
Vancouver, British Columbia

Introduction

THIS IS THE TRUEST BOOK yet written about health in general and diabetes in particular. It deals with a crucial health issue that nearly always gets ignored: the issue of power. Without power, people face more stress and more life conditions that can make them sick. They are less able to take care of themselves, to stay healthy in a toxic environment. And when they do get sick, the medical system reinforces their powerlessness by turning them into "patients," isolating them, piling new demands on them, often making things worse.

Powerlessness has always created illness and medicine has usually failed to respond. There have been exceptions. In 1847, the Berlin City Council sent a young pathologist named Rudolph Virchow to investigate the cause of a typhus outbreak in the province of Upper Silesia (now part of Poland). Virchow concluded that the Council itself had caused the outbreak by its mistreatment of the Silesians. His recommendations included "full democracy for Silesia, making Polish the official language of the region, shifting taxation from the poor to the rich, road construction, and the establishment of farming cooperatives."[1]

The Council didn't like the report, calling it "politics, not medicine." Standing firm, Virchow replied: "Medicine is a social science, and politics nothing but medicine on a grand scale."

Now, 158 years later, Virchow's statement rings truer than ever, and Type 2 diabetes (T2D) is the classic illustration. T2D isn't so much an illness as a racket, foisted on people with less power by those with more power. Rates of T2D are exploding, devastating communities all over the world.

Meanwhile, billions of dollars are being made. Some profit from causing diabetes, others from treating it. Most, at least on the treatment side are doing this with good intentions, but the results are horrifying. Millions of people are getting sick, becoming disabled, dying young. Medicine seems almost completely unable to help, because it doesn't challenge the power relationships that contribute to diabetes and related chronic conditions. Part I of this book describes the social causes of illness and how they make people sick.

In spite of the growing social factors causing illness, there is hope. We can stop the diabetes epidemic, but only if we address the powerlessness and environmental toxicities that cause it. Part II explores a new and better approach to T2D and chronic illness — a social movement approach. Though in its infancy, this movement is gaining momentum. It has started in communities and health care systems, empowering individuals to take care of themselves, strengthening families and encouraging communities to help each other, restructuring health care practices to support healthier living and taking political action to create a healthier environment.

This movement is applicable to more than the way we approach diabetes. Diabetes is not in any way unique among health issues. The same social conditions that cause T2D contribute to most other chronic illnesses — heart disease, asthma, lung disease, arthritis, mental illness, depression, even most forms of cancer. They also promote social problems — crime, drug abuse, family violence — and contribute to terrifying environmental problems such as soil erosion and global warming. The movement spontaneously growing to stop diabetes could benefit a lot of other areas, too.

Coming to the Politics of Health

I have been a nurse for 32 years and have lived with a chronic illness, multiple sclerosis, for 25 years. I specialize in self-care — helping people help themselves. Since the publication of my first book, *The Art of Getting Well: Maximizing Health When You Have a Chronic Illness* (Hunter House, 2002), I've been traveling through the US and England teaching self-care skills and teaching health professionals how to help others succeed at self-care. In my journeys, I have made many remarkable discoveries and met many remarkable people.

Many of these people I worked with, however, didn't make much progress. I met Joan in Omaha, who struggled for years just to get a simple exercise program going. She even had a stationary bike set up in her living room in front of the TV. She never used it. She was too stressed about money to worry about her health. It was only after her money situation improved (by taking in a cousin as a housemate) that she was finally able to start moving.

And for each person who did progress, there were a dozen more in line waiting to fill that place. It seemed self-care could only take you so far, and I wondered why. Seeking out the answers led me to the research and experiences that became *Diabetes: Sugar-Coated Crisis*.

During this time I was lucky to encounter the groundbreaking work of sociologists like Michael Marmot, Leonard Syme and Nancy Adler, who look at health from the perspective of communities, populations and countries. Had I not been searching, I could have worked in clinical medicine all my life and never heard of them. As Dr. Adler says, social medicine and clinical medicine are "separated by a huge gulf. Some of it derives from the difference in focus — clinical medicine focuses on the individual, while public health focuses on populations. Some is difference in thinking style. Some is the overload that physicians feel and resistance to adding something more complicated." A major reason I wrote this book is to try to bridge that gulf.

The sociologists knew what the problem was, but what to do about it? In looking for answers, I came in contact with people who had ideas about possible solutions. At conferences in inner cities and clinics on reservations, I met community leaders, including physicians like America Bracho in Orange County, who demonstrated how people can get healthier by joining forces to change their environment. I met clinicians like Devin Sawyer in Seattle, who showed me how putting people in charge of their own care and bringing them together for mutual support can actually help them overcome diabetes.

I also trained in the programs of Kate Lorig at Stanford and read the books of her associate Albert Bandura, which describe better ways to help people change behavior and gain personal power. I studied the research of psychologist/diabetes educators like William Polonsky and Richard Rubin, who teach what a serious impact life issues have on diabetes and what can be done to deal with these.

I've learned what the barriers are to self-care, and I've learned several ways of getting over those barriers. I learned that people's health flows from the quality and difficulty of their lives. People get sick because their lives are hard, the environment is unhealthy, and they lack the power to respond effectively. Getting better depends on gaining the power to change behavior, environment and lives.

The things I've learned, the people I've met and the efforts being made everywhere in the world to promote health and wellness give me hope, but most of these progressive forces are isolated from one another. I hope this book helps to unite social medicine, clinical medicine and community activism. We need to connect health with other social change movements and use these movements to serve the people who are currently being crushed. At this point, we're losing and diabetes is growing. But I hope that this book will help, and that you will be encouraged to join this movement. You may even realize that you're already part of it.

Prologue: Diabetes 101

READERS WILL NEED TO HAVE a basic understanding of what diabetes is in order to gain the most from the book. If you're already knowledgeable about diabetes, feel free to skip this prologue; otherwise, here is a short, simplified course.

Diabetes is the common name for at least two different diseases. Both result in the body losing part or all of its ability to handle carbohydrates — sugar and foods that break down into sugar. Our bodies need a hormone called insulin to handle sugars, which are our primary source of energy.[1]

Carbohydrates such as breads, cereals, table sugar, pasta or potatoes, when digested, break down into a sugar called glucose. Insulin facilitates the entry of glucose into body cells where it can be used as fuel, or into the liver where it can be stored as starch. Insulin also helps convert extra glucose into fat. Insulin is also necessary for metabolizing other sugars, like milk sugar ("lactose") and fruit sugar ("fructose").

In Type 1 diabetes (T1D), the insulin-producing cells ("beta cells") in the pancreas are damaged or destroyed. There are many causes, but most remain unknown. In the most common type, the diabetic person's own immune system attacks the pancreas and destroys the beta cells. A virus or exposure to chemicals or certain proteins may set off this process. T1D used to be called "juvenile-onset" diabetes, but it can start at any age.

This book deals mostly with Type 2 diabetes (T2D). Most people with T2D still produce insulin but their cells won't cooperate with it. Their muscle and/or liver cells won't absorb the glucose. This is what is known as "insulin resistance." Because the cells don't want any more sugar, glucose builds up in the blood instead and causes problems.

Some of the excess glucose will convert to fat. People with Type 2 often have "metabolic syndrome" or "Syndrome X," symptoms of which can include abdominal fat, high blood pressure, high blood sugar, too much low-density lipoprotein cholesterol (LDL or "bad" cholesterol) and not enough high-density lipoprotein cholesterol (HDL or "good" cholesterol). All of these symptoms are almost certainly related to insulin resistance. T2D used to be called "adult-onset" diabetes, but now is seen in children as young as six.

The pancreas may try to pump out more insulin to overcome the body's insulin resistance. Eventually, though, the beta cells start to wear out, which is when symptoms of diabetes usually become noticeable. Beta cell burnout can be prevented with good self-management and proper care, but most people with Type 2 never get that kind of care.

T2D mostly affects people who are overweight, but that doesn't mean the extra weight is diabetes' major cause. Most heavy people never get diabetes.[2] Quite possibly, various life factors, especially stress and inactivity, cause both the weight gain and the diabetes.

What Diabetes Does

Most people with diabetes live with higher than normal blood sugars. They may feel sluggish and lethargic but have no dramatic symptoms. This could be why at least one third of people with diabetes don't know they have it.

Over time though, these high levels of sugar damage blood vessels, nerves and other organs of the body. This process can lead to complications, including heart attack, stroke, kidney failure, blindness, chronic pain, and loss of feet or legs to amputation. In many communities, diabetes is the leading cause of disability.[3] Diabetes is the fourth leading cause of death in the US and a major contributor to the number one cause — heart disease. Diabetes in the US costs $132 billion a year by official estimates (other estimates are considerably higher).[4] According to the US Centers for Disease Control, 80% of that money is spent on treating complications.[5] Very little is spent on preventing them, says Dr. Jaime Davidson, president of the Endocrine and Diabetes Associates of Texas. An even smaller pittance is spent on preventing diabetes itself, and that amount is decreasing.[6]

Complications can be prevented and often reversed by regulating sugar levels, a feat millions have accomplished through self-care including exercise, stress reduction, a healthy diet, and sometimes medications. It is even possible for people who run high blood sugars to never suffer from serious problems. Other factors besides sugar, such as inflammation, probably contribute to the development of complications.

Doctors call T2D call a "chronic, progressive disease," which translates as you can't get better; the best you can hope for is to slow down the rate of getting worse. This label can make people feel hopeless and out of control, which can lead to stress and ultimately makes the situation worse. In reality, while many patients do get worse over time, some people with T2D do in fact get better. Sometimes they can improve to the point that the usual lab tests reveal no sign of diabetes.[7] Even if people with T2D can't make it go away, they can stabilize their sugars, improve their general health and make some other life changes.

In this way, they can achieve better, healthier lives than they had before.

A person is considered diabetic if their blood sugar is high: a fasting blood sugar (FBS; in Canada this is called an FPG or "fasting plasma glucose") above 126 mg/dl (milligrams per deciliter) on two different occasions or a random glucose above 200 mg/dl. An FBS/FPG between 100–125 mg/dl is classed as "pre-diabetes." Diabetes is usually monitored with an interesting test called a "glycosylated hemoglobin" or "hemoglobin A1C (HgbA1C)." An A1C test measures the percentage of red blood cells that have glucose attached to them. While an FBS or random glucose check only gives a snapshot of a person's sugar level at a particular moment, an A1C reveals how glucose levels have been for the previous 4–8 weeks. A normal A1C is from four to six percent.

A Brief History of Diabetes

As chronic illnesses go, diabetes is relatively new. Arthritis, in contrast, has been around forever. Cavemen had arthritis. Dinosaurs had arthritis.[9] There was no evidence of T2D, though, prior to 10,000 years ago. It started with the rise of agriculture. Hunter-gatherers don't get diabetes, but growing grains and herding animals resulted in the consumption of more calories, more carbohydrates and more saturated fat.

Rich people got more of the food and did less of the work, and a few started to get diabetes. In the 6th Century, three Indian physicians wrote, "Diabetes is the disease of the rich, brought about by overindulgence in oil, flour and sugar."[10] It stayed a rich man's problem until the 20th Century. The poor weren't at risk, because people who eat too few calories rarely get diabetes (although starvation diets — less than 1,000 calories a day — may increase the risk of getting diabetes down the road).

During the world wars, for example, diabetes death rates in Europe dropped by more than half because food was scarce. In modern Haiti, a study found that the poor were eating 980–1,500 calories a day, while the rich were ingesting more than 3,000. Diabetes rates were approximately 100 times higher among the Haitian rich.[11]

T2D rates really took off after the discovery of oil. Oil-powered tractors and reapers allowed farmers to produce huge amounts of grain. Trucks, trains and ships carried these calorie-packed goods all over the country and the world and brought in sugar from the Caribbean and the South. Oil-based fertilizers and chemicals increased food output tremendously. Industrialization, chemical preservation and innovations in packaging allowed for the distribution of richer, unhealthier food, reaching the tables of people who had never had it before.

Now there is so much affordable, accessible food, so much of which is unhealthy, that we have a diabetes pandemic. It's not just food that contributes to the exploding diabetes rates. The "American lifestyle" — car travel replacing bikes and walking, TV watching and sedentary jobs replacing physical activity, high levels of stress, inequality and isolation — also drives diabetes. While technological progress and vast consumption of resources have greatly increased the supply of food and human population numbers, they have not brought greater health, but instead a whole new class of illnesses.

So that's T2D in a nutshell. Obviously, there is a lot more to say about its causes and treatment, and we will. We'll start with who gets T2D and why, who lives well with it and who suffers and how media and mainstream medicine overlook its most important causes and ignore the most promising approaches to dealing with it.

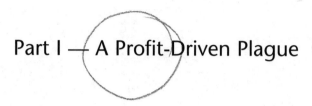

Part I — A Profit-Driven Plague

Diabetes as a Social Disease

*"I guess diabetes is a bunch of family curses,
that is how it started ... Like, my momma had it,
father got it, and you know, all of us just
got a curse on us. If it runs in your family,
you will wind up getting it"*

— MONIQUE, AGE 48, CHARLESTON, SOUTH CAROLINA

"If we do not know our history, we believe it is our fate."

— HANNAH ARENDT

A TIDAL WAVE, A FLOOD of diabetes is sweeping over the world. It afflicts about 200 million people, an increase of almost 400% in the last 30 years.[1] It cripples communities. It bankrupts health care systems. About 10 million people a year die from it (more than from AIDS). It's getting worse: about 400 million more are pre-diabetic, on their way to full-blown illness.

And they are blamed for it. Most doctors and health writers will tell you that Type 2 diabetes (90% of all cases) is a genetic curse, the result of bad behavior, or some combination of the two. The blame for diabetes falls entirely on the person who has it. Either you're doing something wrong or there's something wrong *with* you.[2]

But diabetes is not something people do to themselves and it's not a curse. It's not something that just happens. T2D is a social disease — not social in the sense of "sexually transmitted," but in the reality that society itself has the disease. Individuals get the symptoms and pay the price, but the environment is set up to make people sick. It's toxically high in sugar and stress, low in social support, opportunities to exercise or to feel good about ourselves. The unhealthy state of the environment in modern society will give people diabetes if they lack the power to fight it off or change it.

As with any flood, it's the people of the lowlands who get the wettest. In the developed world, it's the people lowest on the social and economic ladder, the ones with the least power, who make up the majority of diabetics and suffer the most complications.[3] In the developing world, the very poorest, those who get little food and rely on walking as their only means of transportation, don't get much diabetes, but those somewhat higher on the economic chain do.

In addition to affecting the poor communities where it indeed does the most damage, the diabetes flood reaches far beyond. As an old African saying goes, "When it's raining in the valley, it's snowing on the mountain." All over the world, indigenous people, people of color and poor people are drowning in a toxic sea of sugar, stress, inactivity and inequality. But the same poisoned environment puts people of all classes and colors at varying degrees of risk for diabetes.

If T2D is a social disease, you wouldn't expect medical care to be effective against it, and you would be right. In the US, we have a two trillion dollar medical system that ignores the social causes of illness. Instead, it focuses almost entirely on genetics, biochemistry and other avenues that lead to drug therapy as the

primary solutions. These therapies don't work very well; no diabetes drug except possibly insulin is as effective as exercise.
They distract from what really works — building capacity for
self-care, empowering communities and creating a healthier environment. To see how skewed the mainstream approach to
T2D is, let's take a quick trip to the Arizona desert.

"The Most Studied People in the World"

Ground Zero of the diabetes epidemic is in Southern Arizona's
Sonora Desert, near the Gila River. The Pima Indians, or the
A'a'tam a'kimult, which means "River People," have a rate of
T2D as high as 70% among adults, the highest in the world (although some Pacific Islanders are catching up). These numbers
have brought carloads of scientists to the Pima's beautiful
desert home. Western science hopes to better understand diabetes by focusing on the sickest people. Millions of dollars have
been spent. In the words of Dr. Ann Bullock, medical director
of the Cherokee Health and Medical Division in North Carolina, the Pima are "among the most studied people in the world."

But it's mostly wasted effort, because they're looking in the
wrong place — at the patients, not at the environment. Of
around 500 published Pima/diabetes studies indexed on Pub-
Med, the US government's medical research database, more
than 60% focus on genetics. Most of the others deal with connections between genes and body chemistry. Only a handful
concern treatment, and only three focus on behavior change.
None deal with the Pima's history, economy or the cultural
strains they are under.

Way down the line, this genetic research could possibly lead
to some new drug therapies, maybe even some that are slightly
better than what we have now. Somebody may make a lot of
money. But it certainly won't do anything to help the Pima or
others in their situation, because it doesn't address the real,
social causes of their health crisis.

Of course, genes are important, but their role is often misunderstood. As Matt Ridley explains in his book, *Nature via Nurture,* genes interact with the environment. They are turned on and off and their functions are modified by their environment and by parents' and grandparents' environments. You can't understand genes or illness without connecting them to the environment.[4]

It is highly misleading to say that the Pima have an unusual genetic risk for diabetes. Before the Europeans came, diabetes was virtually unknown among Native Americans. There is no word for diabetes in most traditional Native languages. Even in 1933, Dr. Hancock of the Indian Health Service reported seeing exactly one case of diabetes among Native Americans in two years of work in Arizona.[5] If you look at pictures from the early 20th Century, the Pima aren't overweight. They are athletic. They are graceful, beautiful. And Pima in Mexico, who have the same genes but live a more traditional lifestyle, have low rates of diabetes, similar to their non-Pima neighbors.[6]

What the Pima have is an intolerance of the modern American way of life — especially the concentrated carbohydrates and the lack of physical activity — and a history of trauma most of us couldn't imagine. What they have is a lack of power. The American diet (and a very poor version of it at that) was imposed on the Pima at the same time as they lost their land, their freedom and their way of life. For 2,000 years, they had been successful farmers, hunters and weavers. In 1928, the construction of the Coolidge Dam diverted their water supply, and much of their traditional means of living went with it.[7] They became much less physically active or economically viable. Their culture was suppressed and many families broken up under government programs to raise Native children in boarding schools.

For this genocidal trauma, they were compensated with high-sugar, high-fat welfare food and access to television, a trade that has been forced on conquered people all over the world. You lose your self-determination, your culture, your job and your hope, but you do get TV, Big Macs, Cokes and Type 2 Diabetes.

Few people have genes strong enough to protect against the kinds of injuries that the Pima have suffered. Few could cope with such a toxic physical and psychological environment. All those injuries have direct physical effects. They cause insulin resistance and high blood pressure. They make it more difficult to live a healthy life or find reasons to do so.

True Causes of T2D

The Pima are an extreme case but they're not unique. Many people with diabetes or pre-diabetes have experienced these kinds of injuries, although usually to a lesser degree. In the US and Canada, most Native nations, most people of African ancestry and many Latino communities have faced such historical trauma. They have very high diabetes rates, as do some low-income Whites and American Southerners. T2D can be a very accurate gauge of where a group ranks in society. In general, the less power, money and status a group has, the more T2D they will have.[8]

The same is true for individuals.[9] Having less money leads to a greater risk of diabetes. Less education leads to more diabetes. There seems to be a direct correlation between unemployment and diabetes. All these things are aspects of having little power. Trauma can also rob you of power by damaging your self-confidence and taking away your sense of safety.[10] Being an abused child or growing up in an insecure home, or the death, jailing or substance abuse problem of a parent, can put you at risk for diabetes.[11] Soldiering is often traumatic and predicts diabetes. Military veterans have more than twice the diabetes rates of non-veterans.[12]

The pathways from difficult lives to diabetes are still being explored, but stress and powerlessness play major roles. Chronic stress contributes to diabetes directly through the action of stress hormones and indirectly through its effect on behaviors. Stress is not evenly distributed through society:

people with less power have more stress. Chapter 2 explains these effects in detail.

Stress isn't the whole story, of course. The availability of healthy food and opportunities to exercise play a big role, as do motivational factors such as self-confidence, positive goals and reasons to live. The effects of the social environment on diabetes are far stronger than any known gene or behavior, as the experience of two tribes in Southern California will show.

Genes and the Casino

In the dry, gentle hills of Southern California's Riverside and San Bernardino counties live two bands of the Cuahuilla Nation, the Morongo and the Torrez-Martinez.[13] They come from the same stock and have lived near each other and intermarried for hundreds of years, creating a common gene pool. Neither band gets much exercise. Their diabetes rates should be similar. But, based on health provider estimates, the Torrez-Martinez have almost four times the diabetes rate of the Morongo. How can this be?

The difference is that the Morongo have a successful casino. While the Torrez-Martinez live in trailers in a desert far from the road, have no money and near-total unemployment, the Morongo have some hope. With a casino, they can send their kids to college, get jobs and buy trucks. As the largest employer for the nearby town of Banning, they are an important part of society. They have the same genes as the Torrez-Martinez but a different amount of power and different resources. (It must be said that, while neither tribe eats a particularly healthy diet, the Morongo get more steak and eggs, while the Torrez-Martinez eat more tortillas, beans and rice. This may account for some of the diabetes difference, but the protein intake, too, is related to their economic status.)

Genes haven't changed much in the 30 years of the diabetes epidemic. Neither the indigenous people nor anyone else has suddenly turned into a gang of gluttonous hogs, eating themselves to death. What has changed is the environment around food and physical activity. As Dr. Gabor Maté, author of *When The Body Says No,* puts it, blaming people's genes for their problems "allows us to avoid disturbing questions about the nature of the society in which we live."[14]

People used to think tuberculosis was some kind of inherited weakness.[15] But when housing improved and poverty decreased, TB became much less common, and when some moderately effective drugs were discovered, TB nearly disappeared in rich countries. Most likely, genes play a larger role in diabetes than they do in TB, but with positive environmental change, Type 2 diabetes could disappear, too. But that will require a different kind of medicine, one that looks at changing social environments, not just individual behaviors.

Doing It to Themselves?

Most people are only dimly aware of the connection between environment, behavior and health, if they recognize it at all. Recently, I was telling a lawyer acquaintance about the social causes of diabetes over a healthy salad-bar lunch at a trendy restaurant overlooking the San Francisco beachfront. He didn't want to hear it. "All they have to do is stop eating," he said. "All they have to do is go to the gym. What's so hard about that?"

It's a common response — those who don't blame genes, blame behavior. And behavior *is* important. People who eat right, exercise and relax will probably be healthier, no matter what genes they have or how much stress they're under. In our society, however, powerful social forces block physical activity and lead to unmanageable levels of stress. Huge corporations work very hard to ensure that we eat lots of unhealthy food. Economic and social demands limit the time, money and energy we can put into self-care. Many of us, especially those with little power, carry burdens of emotional pain and anxiety that are easily treated with sugar. We learn unhealthy behaviors before we know better, often before we can speak. And we maintain those behaviors because our environment is set up to maintain them.

T2D, heart disease and other chronic conditions are often called "lifestyle illnesses." This is wrong. It's not "lifestyles;" it's the difficult lives those behaviors are in. Poor people have worse health and worse health behaviors, so people think the health problems come from the behaviors. But careful studies show that less than 30% (as low as 12% in some studies) of all the excess illness among low-income people comes from behaviors like smoking, drinking, overeating or not exercising. Stress and the environment appear to play much bigger parts.[16,17]

Social Diseases Need Social Approaches

Healthier behaviors around food, exercise and relaxation are crucial to leading a healthy life, and they are possible, but only with sufficient support. People get sick because of their social conditions. So we need a social approach, the power of people working together to change those conditions and get well. The elements of the social approach are:

- Building personal power — self-confidence, self-esteem, positive goals and reasons to live.
- Building social power — working together in families, communities, support groups and other collectives.
- Changing the environment — starting with the individual home, to the community, to the larger society.

This is a public health approach and is practically unknown to modern medicine. Nearly all doctors prefer to treat patients one by one. They prescribe drugs and behaviors and hope for the best. Patients rarely get the best results, because the drugs are not very effective, and because patients have too many other demands to succeed at behavior change and too few internal and external resources to cope with their environment.

Looking at one person at a time, we can see only genes and behavior. These factors are important, but when we look at diabetes in groups and communities, we can see causes and cures that may have remained invisible at the individual level. We can see ways forward for people who, as individuals, seemed blocked.

The Power of the Social Approach

How many people have started exercise programs but haven't stayed with them? An individual regime that relies only on individual willpower is difficult to maintain and often results in giving up. Taking a social approach to exercise reduces obstacles, makes for greater motivation and a stronger chance of sticking to it. Social approaches could include anything from finding one regular exercise partner, to going to a gym with built-in support like a family YMCA or Curves,[18] to church-based exercise programs, to attending martial arts classes at your local hospital. Some communities take social exercise even farther, like the Seattle community that has set up a senior/teen joint walking program, or the Alaska Natives who have re-discovered traditional sports to inspire people to keep active, or the establishment of community safety walks in communities where people are not comfortable walking alone.

Similar creative solutions are being conceived for healthy eating and stress reduction. Possibly even greater results come from working to change the social environment, such as communities fighting for employment opportunities for youth, or the transformation of local schools into community centers where whole families can participate in education (and sometimes exercise).

Health care providers can and should employ the power of social support in the form of group appointments, classes led by people with diabetes, support groups and mentor programs.

These kinds of inspiring programs, have been successfully implemented around the world. Research shows they work, and you will read about them in Chapter 7 and 8.

Shame as a Health Hazard

Why are the social causes of diabetes important to know? When people are blamed for their own illness, they often become ashamed or fatalistic, and these feelings can sap their ability to change behaviors and to take care of themselves. Most people with diabetes rarely talk about it, even with other diabetics. They may consider it too shameful or a sign of weakness. I interviewed 30 people with T2D for this book, and only a few had told their friends that they had it. Some even swore me to secrecy. They mistook lack of social power for personal weakness. To remedy these feelings of shame and helplessness, it is important for people to understand their social environment and its direct effect on their health.

Oklahoma Native American diabetes therapist Regina Whitewolf can sympathize with these feelings. "My Dad was a national tribal leader," she says. "He worked with hundreds of tribes. My mother said, 'your Dad has diabetes and he doesn't want anyone to know.' And we never talked about it ever. He died at 58. When I was diagnosed with diabetes, I said, 'This is crazy.' We need to talk about these things. We have to share."

When whole communities are sick, they may feel hopeless and take it out on each other. As Whitewolf says, "we're oppressive to each other because it's safer than dealing with the people who have done this to us." This kind of transference — inflicting anger on those who don't deserve it, including ourselves — doesn't apply only to indigenous people. How many people become self-destructive or attack their loved ones over their problems, either because they don't know that there are social causes to these problems or, if they do, because they feel those causes are too powerful to face?

This pattern of blame and shame creates formidable barriers, which cripple efforts at personal or community health. Learning about social causes and adopting social approaches can remove the guilt and give people the strength to make changes in their lives. It's quite possible that when people come together around health issues, they will be a force that can heal the unhealthy environment. One person taking care of him/herself can inspire many more. Groups working together — families, neighbors, churches, unions, community groups or any people with shared interests and needs — can inspire individuals to care for themselves and help create better social environments. And who knows where that kind of movement will lead?

How to Use This Book

This book does *not* claim to teach the details of diabetes self-care, although I have included a one-chapter "Self-Care Appendix," at the back. By reading this book you will get an understanding of the social dynamics of health that will help you deal with diabetes or any chronic condition. If, however, you have T2D and want to learn more after reading the Appendix, the resource list gives some very informative books and web sites. You may also want to get more information from a health professional or skilled lay diabetes worker.

Some of the ideas in this book may seem radical or difficult to accept, but they are all backed by solid science and explained in clear, understandable terms. It may be more scientific than you want: feel free to skip parts that don't appeal to you. If you are interested doing further research or checking the data, see the Notes and Resource List section at the back. For the moment I want to take you on a tour of the toxic environment, starting with an exploration of stress as you've probably never understood it before.

Chapter 2

Toxic Environment: Stress and Inequality

W HILE THE "AMERICAN LIFESTYLE," chock full of fat, sugar, cars and television and addressed in detail in Chapter 3, encourages diabetes all over the world, Chapter 2 asks why some groups are afflicted so much more than others. And why, within these groups, do some individuals and families become overweight, and suffer diabetes and other diseases, while a family down the block remains healthy? As we know, the usual explanations involve genetics and behavior, but this chapter presents other causes — stress, inequality and lack of power.

Stress is a major contributor to diabetes, and power is its most important treatment. Stress, sometimes called the "fight or flight" response, tells the liver and other cells to release stored glucose into the blood so the muscles and brain can use it for action. Cortisol, the main stress hormone, increases insulin resistance in both the muscles and the liver.[1] Under stress, only the muscles actually being used for fighting or running will open to insulin and the glucose it's carrying. Other body tissues resist the insulin, so the vital muscles can have more fuel.

But in modern society, common causes of stress aren't due to predatory threats, as in the wild, meaning there is usually no physical response, no fight or flight. You just sit there and worry. The lethal combination of stress and physical inactivity results in the extra sugar staying in the blood or turning into abdominal fat.[2] If stress is chronic, insulin resistance builds, leading to eventual weight gain and T2D.

Stress hormones also increase blood pressure and heart rate in preparation for immediate action. It is a survival mechanism designed for fleeing a hungry lion or fighting a dangerous enemy. Stress doesn't care about our long-term health, because there will be no long-term if we don't survive the immediate threat. Stress has no use for the immune system, the body's self-repair and disease-fighting program; repair can wait until the crisis is over.[3]

But for people with little power, the crisis is never over. So over time, chronic stress is like endlessly deferring maintenance on your car. Like your car, your body will tend to break down if maintenance (the immune system) is suppressed. If you have stress and diabetes, high sugar levels will damage blood vessels, and because the normal repair systems aren't working, blood vessels will have a hard time trying to restore themselves.

Stress can also cause T2D indirectly through behaviors, because we tend to react to stress by consuming sugar and fat. These "comfort foods" raise levels of serotonin and endorphin, chemicals that make us feel more in control and less overwhelmed.[4] I'll describe the psychological effects of food in depth in Chapter 3.

The healthy way to respond to stress is through physical activity, similar to the way animals react when threatened by a predator. Activity burns up the sugar and restores the hormonal balance, reducing feelings of stress. But in the modern environment it's difficult to react to stress this way. Society sets up our lives to make us passive.

Power and Stress

Power is the antidote to stress. Drs. Daniel Cox and Linda Gonder-Frederick, of the University of Virginia Health Science Center define stress as "the adaptation process to events (stressors) which threaten disruption to an organism's homeostasis."[4] "Homeostasis" is our bodies' physical balance; disrupting homeostasis means threatening life itself. Stress occurs when perceived threats reach beyond our perceived ability to control them. Under stress, we feel that most of our energy is going towards trying to cope, just trying to keep our heads above water, an image that captures the feeling of stress very well.

It's not easy to capture this kind of stress in a controlled experiment. We're not talking about a busy day at work or the kids getting into a fight when you're trying to cook dinner or trying to solve math problems with bad music playing in a psychology lab. These kinds of stresses don't have a significant impact on blood sugars. But living with the threat of violence, job stresses beyond control, economic insecurity, dealing every day with racism, sexism or other prejudices,[5] caring for a demented parent, feeling hopeless or useless, lonely, unloved or uncared for, stresses like these can wear a body down and predispose you to conditions like T2D, as well as and heart disease and many others.

There is a direct correlation between stress and lack of power. Because stress results when life's dangers and demands exceed your power to control them, *the less power you have, the more stress you will have.* Imagine walking down the street and meeting a hungry, man-eating lion. You would be highly stressed. But if you were riding down the same street in an Abrams tank and met that same lion, you likely wouldn't be stressed at all. You'd be safe, and you might have a "cute lion" story to tell at work. When you have the power to cope easily, there is no stress.

Access to money, a source of power, can reduce stress. Let's say my company was planning to send my job to Bangladesh. If I had a million dollars in the bank, I wouldn't feel stressed. The job loss could potentially hurt emotionally, but it probably wouldn't affect my health. And if I felt I could easily find another job, it would be even less stressful. But if I lived paycheck to paycheck and believed that getting another job would be very difficult, and had a family depending on my income, worrying about the job loss might not only keep me up at night, but keep my blood sugar levels up too, even if the threatened move never happened. My body would be screaming, "Run! Fight! Climb a tree or something," but I couldn't. And I would pay a price that could eventually include T2D.

Love and self-confidence can build power and reduce stress. Say the Bangladesh scenario has played out, and the pressure of unemployment has me considering taking up smoking again. A close, supportive family that encourages me to start fresh while keeping my behavior in check could reduce my stress dramatically. If, on the other hand, my family is more critical than supportive, if I have few friends or am totally alone, I might be far more likely to smoke, drink or binge on chocolate cake — all of which are easily accessible stress relievers.

Some of us figuratively ride in tanks while others scrounge transfers to pay bus fare. Some have big bank accounts while others lack lunch money, and some of us have close, supportive families, while others are isolated. So some of us have a lot more stress than others, and the high-stress group tends to also have a lot of health and life problems, as the following research shows.

The Health "Gradient"

Until about 20 years ago, scientists thought that the difference in health between rich and poor was simply a question of deprivation. If you are very poor, you will of course have health problems that better off people don't. But in the 1980's, British studies proved that lower socio-economic status (SES) leads to worse health, all the way from the bottom of society to the top.[6] Even doctors and lawyers had worse health than the few people who ranked above them. Clearly, poverty and deprivation were not the cause of this disparity. Access to medical care had nothing to do with it either, because in England, everyone has similar care, and it's free.

So what causes this "gradient" in health? Michael Marmot and his associates have found that the main causes are factors related to stress — anxiety, depression, trauma, economic difficulties — and power/protection — education, self-confidence and social support. People with less power tend to have more of the stress-related factors and fewer of the protective ones.

The Stress of Looking Up

If you don't believe having less power is stressful, check your blood pressure the next time a cop stops you or your boss yells at you. Blood pressure is highly variable. It rises when a person is talking with someone more powerful than they are.[7] In some people, blood pressure rises during a visit to the doctor's office. This is called "white-coat hypertension." (The white coats are the lab coats worn by the doctors and nurses.) Because of this tendency, doctors may think these patients have high blood pressure (hypertension), when they actually have normal pressure most of the time. This increase is part of the stress reaction; being around powerful people is stressful. (Note that high blood pressure is often a warning of coming diabetes.)[8]

For people with less power, it can seem that everyone they meet is wearing a white coat. This situation applies to many people of color. It also describes the experience of millions of others, such as low-wage workers, people who are overweight or people who are disabled. Even people with none of these disadvantages can feel powerless if they have been neglected or traumatized. And if most people are more powerful than you, you will experience stress most of the time, and you will be at risk for hypertension, heart disease, and diabetes.

It's natural to stress out when you have less power. Throughout history, for both humans and animals, having less power has meant you were likely to get physically attacked. In modern society, the attacks are usually not physical — they're economic or emotional — but they still hurt. Like primates, people are always checking to see where we rank, to avoid battles that we know we cannot win.[9] This checking is usually subconscious; we don't know we are doing it, but it stresses us, affects our behavior and raises our blood pressures and sugars just the same.

This is probably why the more unequal a society is, the worse its overall health is likely to be. This has been demonstrated by dozens of studies cited by Richard Wilkinson in his book *Unhealthy Societies*.[10] Life expectancies and health outcomes are best in Scandinavia and Japan, where income inequality is least. Cubans (living in a relatively equal society) have an average life expectancy essentially the same as Americans do, even though Cuba's average income is far lower, and Cubans spend only 4% as much on health care as Americans do.[11] In explaining the average level of health, the overall wealth or poverty of a society is not as important as the degree of inequality, once a certain threshold of wealth is reached. (The most destitute countries do have the worst health.)

"Low status stress" is everywhere in modern society. Every school and workplace has ranking systems. Some are formal, like job titles and awards. Other pecking orders, like the "popular kids" in high school, are less formal, but still powerful. But low status is just one source of stress.

No Stress Like Economic Stress

We have an image of stress as resulting from a very busy life. The phones are ringing, we're racing around town; we've got deadlines, high noise levels and not enough time. All the little crises of life add up to this feeling we call "stress." While extreme busyness is one cause of stress, it's not the only one or the worst one.

More damaging than busy stress is economic stress, not having a secure job, not knowing if you can make ends meet from month to month. This kind of stress eats at you day and night, raising the body's cortisol levels. A high proportion of people with little money, insecure housing, unpaid bills or temporary jobs, have Type 2 diabetes or pre-diabetes.

The stress of low status and a low income can actually be seen in the body. For example, poor people's adrenal glands (which respond to stress) are often bigger than those of people who are better off. But rich people's thymus glands (which help the body repair itself and fight infections) are usually bigger than those of the poor.[12] The higher day-to-day stress of being poor saps the energy needed for repair, and the thymus gland shrinks.

Economic stress can also damage our social lives, which leads to even further stress. A peaceful, loving, supportive home can protect against stress, but it's difficult to maintain such a home when you're worried about being evicted from it. Studies of child abuse show that the biggest risk factors for abuse are marital problems, unemployment and debt.[13] And being abused as a child is a risk factor for Type 2 diabetes. So economic stress can undermine the social support we need to deal with life.

Stress Starts Early

How do people get stressed? It usually starts early, sometimes even before birth. A highly stressed mother tends to give birth to an easily stressed child.[15] Parental stress and early childhood experiences can leave people with a lifetime inheritance of stress, if something isn't done to heal it.

Rat[14, 16] and primate (monkey and ape)[15, 17] studies show that animals raised without much parental stroking and support are much more sensitive to stress. They overreact to small problems and suffer heart disease and other stress-related illnesses at a much higher rate. We see exactly the same patterns among humans. Kids who get less positive attention from parents and other adults tend to have more reactive stress systems and consequently more disease.

Depression and Power

Depression is the leading cause of disability in the US,[18] but most people don't know that it's an entirely normal response to lack of power. Paul Gilbert, author of *Overcoming Depression,* explains that depressed people present themselves as "downcast, unchallenging and unthreatening." This behavior might save your life, if it keeps you out of fights where you would likely get clobbered. Imagine you're one of the weaker chimps in the troop, and any chimp you argue with is going to kick your butt. That would be depressing, but the depression might keep your bones from getting broken.

Take this one step further. If being depressed — sad, quiet, "unchallenging" — keeps you out of trouble, how about being fat? What about being sick? What about sitting in front of the TV all day? Those will keep you on the sidelines: feeling helpless, hopeless, frustrated maybe, but safe. What about having high blood sugar? That will make you tired and dragged out, and no threat to anyone.

Depression may be protective, but it's stressful. It feels awful, and sugar is one of the most reliable ways to feel better. So depression can lead to diabetes through stress or diet. Or through lack of exercise, because depression makes you want to stay in bed, preferably stay in bed and eat donuts. Many times, depression and diabetes represent two aspects of the same disease, called by the names insulin resistance, metabolic syndrome, or powerlessness.

The Impact of Trauma

A history of trauma is associated with diabetes. After trauma, people's stress levels, if not treated, can remain high until they die or their adrenals burn out.[19] This may be one reason why military veterans have such a high rate of diabetes.

Traumatized parents tend to produce traumatized children. Native Americans, African-Americans and others who have suffered historical traumas like genocide and slavery may live in a state of PTSD (post-traumatic stress disorder) their whole lives, and that stress gets passed down for generations if there is no action to relieve it. The Cherokee's history provides a good illustration. First, European germs wiped out half the population. They were then rounded up and forced out of their Georgia homes on the Trail of Tears.[20] Another 4,000 people, including most of the elders, died on this 1,000-mile forced winter march to Oklahoma. Finally, their children were kidnapped and sent to boarding schools, forbidden to speak their own language or see their families. Many were frequently beaten and even sexually abused.[21]

But the Trail of Tears ended in 1839. How could this trauma be causing diabetes today? People, like the Cherokee, who live with high levels of grief, anger, fear, shame and stress, will often act self-destructively or violently, piling new layers of trauma on their children. The dominant group in society may continue inflicting violence, discrimination and high levels of unemployment, adding to the stress of those who live under them. This trauma builds up over time instead of abating, and puts those suffering it at risk for diabetes and other conditions.

A big part of recovery from trauma is changing or escaping the situation where the trauma occurred. Look at the history of the Jewish and Armenian survivors of genocide. Some of those families came to North America or other hospitable countries and starting doing much better economically and socially. Generally, these parents did not pass trauma onto their children.

But many First Nations people, especially on the reservations, live in the same places where the trauma happened, under the control of people much like the people who inflicted it on them. It is very difficult — though not by any means impossible — to heal trauma in this situation. Many practitioners believe that undergoing therapy for trauma and PTSD does help people cope with historical trauma, especially if social conditions improve.

Most African-Americans are descendants of people traumatized by slavery, and many families have gone through 140 years of trauma since — arrests, violence, discrimination. Many immigrants and children of immigrants lived the trauma of being left at home while parents emigrated, and discriminated against once they got where they were going. Those who live around violence, in or out of their homes, are also at risk of becoming traumatized. But even the seemingly less major problems, those that don't affect entire groups of people but are more immediate to the individual, such as losing your job or your home, having a family member arrested or on drugs, breaking up of a marriage through divorce or death, any of these can be a form of trauma.

Like depression, trauma can create diabetes through a stress response or through behavior that stems from trying to cope with it. To deal with it, most people need both professional help and the support of others. Improving lives tends to relieve trauma, so improving the condition of a community can often significantly heal traumatic stress for individuals in that community.

Deprivation

The most obvious (but not the most common) way that powerlessness makes people sick is deprivation or relative poverty. People may not have access to healthy food or may not be able to afford it. Some people may not have access to medical care.

Some can't afford medications or diabetes testing equipment. Even people with medical insurance often can't afford dental care. This can be a serious problem in diabetes, as gum infections make diabetes worse, and vice versa.[22]

Stress can be physical as well as emotional. Cold, heat, or fatigue are stressful and can impact diabetes. Infections are a source of stress and raise blood sugars. Chronic infections such as dental and skin problems can make diabetes control nearly impossible. And who is most likely to have such problems?

Sometimes the pure difficulty of survival impedes living a healthy life. If you have to work two jobs to keep a roof over your head, it may be hard to find energy to exercise. If you live in a war zone, with bullets flying outside and angry words inside, it may be difficult to relax. Letting kids out to play may seem too dangerous, no matter how much they need the exercise.

Deprivation may include lack of clean water and air, leading to exposure to toxic chemicals. Vietnam veterans who develop diabetes can claim it as a service-related illness. That's because Agent Orange, the herbicide used in the Vietnam War, is now known to cause diabetes.[23] Although Agent Orange isn't used anymore, other chemicals in the same class are still being produced and sold. Those who live near the chemical factories or work in the fields might absorb some of those chemicals. There may be toxic substances in food, water, and air, or in building materials and cleaning chemicals. More research is needed, but studies have found a strong correlation between air pollution and diabetes.[24]

The Future of Stress

If we want to stop diabetes, stress reduction and stress management need to be important parts of medical management and self-care efforts. They need to be practiced by individuals, groups and communities. Medical systems must treat stress and depression as primary aspects of treatment, not "alternative" or "complementary" add-ons.

Unless we make major social changes, the stress in people's lives is quite likely to get worse. The more unequal a society is, the more status-related stress it will have. So current economic policies in the US and many other countries almost guarantee that the rates of stress-related illness such as T2D and heart disease will soar in coming years. Fighting for more equality is a long-term solution, and may even help in the short term by making us feel useful and providing a sense of hope.

Acknowledging lack of power doesn't mean accepting it forever. By understanding power dynamics, we can act to improve health and entire lives and perhaps start to equalize power relationships. But in understanding diabetes, we also need to know why our food and activity environments are so unhealthy, which we will explore in the next chapter.

Chapter 3

Toxic Environment:
Food and Inactivity

*"Toxic is a strong word, but powerful language is needed to describe
the situation. [Unhealthy food] is accessible 24 hours per day,
is cheap, promoted heavily, served in huge portions,
designed to taste good and keep people coming back for more."*

— KELLY BROWNELL, PH.D., FOOD FIGHT

IN CHAPTER 2, we saw how stress and lack of power contribute to diabetes. But those mind/body factors are only half the story. Environments loaded with fat, sugar, and barriers to exercise are equally important. This chapter looks at the food and exercise aspects of modern environments, how they came to be so toxic and the debilitating effect they have on people.

Living on the Feedlot

On Route 63 in the low hills of eastern Nebraska, near the town of Ashland, a small cattle ranch straddles the road. On one side, young animals walk around freely, eating green grass in the warm spring sunshine. When they reach a certain age, though, they are moved across the road into a dirt pen for fattening.

Fenced in with dozens of other steers, they have nowhere to go and nothing to do except eat.

Two large food troughs run all the way across the pen. They are filled with concentrated carbohydrates in the form of grain and a mash of animal byproducts and chemicals.[1] The animals have no way to resist the excess food and no reason to do so. They have no way to escape and no way to change their environment.

If you added a couple of large TV sets and some video games, the feedlot wouldn't be that different from many human environments. Consider housing projects, call centers or office "cube farms." Many people go from home feedlots to work and school lots, traveling in mobile lots called cars. Others don't even have that many places to go. They have few opportunities to move or connect with nature, lots of stress and not much to look forward to.

But they do have a lot of food. Much of it is processed grain and meat products, better tasting versions of what the cattle eat. The fact is that society places millions of people in environments like those used for cattle, *and for many of the same reasons*. Feedlots serve two purposes. They make cattle grow faster and fatter for less money than it costs to raise cattle that graze on grass. Feedlots also make cattle easier to control. Now, nobody is fattening people for slaughter. But some people benefit from having us consume more stuff, whether it's food or other products and services.

If you don't have time or energy to move around, or interesting things to do, you will certainly consume more. If you are depressed or stressed, you will be tempted to eat sweet and fat foods that make you feel good. And if you get an illness like diabetes, you will consume a whole range of new, very expensive products to treat it or live with it.

Besides, people are easier to control if they're out of shape, fat, and sick. Nobody causes trouble when their blood sugars are up. We don't feel up to it. This sickening effect may not be intentional, and the food industry may not acknowledge it, even to themselves. It's probably just a side effect of companies doing what makes money, but when there's a tidal wave of diabetes washing over you, it may help to know where it's coming from.

Who's Running the Ranch?

How did the food environment we live in get so unhealthy? For one thing, our food, like cattle feed, got much more calorie concentrated. With the development of mechanized, petrochemical agriculture, producers had more grains than they could profitably sell. So they started feeding it to animals (like on the feedlots) and started processing it into sweet, calorie-rich foods, which became widely available and were shipped all over the world.

In the 1970s, Japanese scientists found a way to make corn into a sweetener called high-fructose corn syrup (HFCS).[2] HFCS is six times sweeter than table sugar. Now most packaged foods, especially soda pop, contain it, and it adds hundreds of calories a day to the diets of Americans and people who eat like them. About the same time, engineers figured out how to make palm oil — a vegetable oil that is fattier and cheaper than most animal fats — into a useful food additive. Both HFCS and palm oil give packaged food a long shelf life as well as a good taste, appearance and feel, at the slight cost of a variety of health concerns, including overweight and T2D.

Cheap, tasty, corporate-produced and attractively packaged foods are available everywhere. Soft drinks are sold in schools, gas stations, even hospitals. Hamburger chains have huge advertising budgets. When was the last time you saw an ad for a vegetable? If money is no object, if you have good food information and enough time, if fruits and vegetables are locally available, and your health is more important to you than a dozen other, more immediate demands, you can eat a healthy diet. Otherwise, it's hard.

Politics and Subsidies

I'm not alleging that anyone is intentionally giving people diabetes. But the food industry knows that what they're doing is, at the very least, making people fat, and despite this awareness, they don't stop. Instead, they have aggressively blocked efforts to get people to eat better.[3]

When the World Health Organization developed some reasonable food guidelines advising people to eat less sugar, "the United States Department of Health and Human Services should have applauded," say nutrition scientists Kelly Brownell, Ph.D., and Marion Nestle, Ph.D. "Instead it produced a 28-page, line-by-line critique. Much evidence argues [that this was] blatant pandering to American food companies that produce much of the world's high-calorie, high-profit sodas and snacks, especially the makers of sugars, the main ingredients in many of these products."[4]

The food industry has also introduced bills in state legislatures and congress to ban lawsuits against restaurants and food manufacturers for contributing to obesity.[5] They have gotten the federal government to censor ads promoting breastfeeding over bottle-feeding.[6] They have enforced "pouring contracts" with school districts.[7] These contracts give particular beverage companies exclusive rights to sell canned and bottled drinks in schools. Pepsi has sued to enforce these contracts, in one case suing students who tried to sell bottled water to raise funds for school sports.[8]

To be fair, food companies do sponsor physical activity programs in communities and schools. In this way, they gain good publicity for themselves and deflect criticism of their food marketing practices. But they're still good programs.

One of the largest and richest companies is ADM, Archer Daniels Midland, which calls itself "supermarket to the world."

Their sales in fiscal 2003 were over $30 billion! Most of their products are grains and sugars, and many are highly subsidized by the federal government. Subsidies to US sugar growers have led to ecological disasters. One example is in Florida, where the Everglades National Park lost most of its water to irrigators growing surplus sugar. According to James Brovey of the Cato Institute, "these subsidies have cost American taxpayers and consumers billions of dollars."[9] The health effects are even more significant. Governments subsidize fast-food start-ups through small business and minority-owned business assistance. Government subsidies for unhealthy food are an important piece of the diabetes epidemic.

Feedlots for Humans

When I thought of the analogy between feedlots and human environments, I ran it by some veterinary science professors at the University of California at Davis. Professor John Maas wrote me a thoughtful e-mail of disagreement, explaining the differences. His concern was that I was too hard on the feedlots; in his view, they are healthier than human environments! The cattle's food is scientifically formulated, he said, and their body fat increase from the fields to the feedlot is only 5% or so.

They may also be less stressed than we are. Another professor, Jim Reynolds, told me about his visits to the cattle. "They look pretty happy," he said. "They're group animals, and they're in a group. Well-run feedlots don't overcrowd them, because you don't want to have more animals than can walk up and eat at the same time."

They are even protected from steer-on-steer violence. "There are cowboys who go through the lot and take out the dominant animals," says Reynolds, "because otherwise they would push the other ones around and keep them from eating. That potential stressor is removed. We humans certainly live much more stressful lives than the livestock."

Of course, not all feedlots are well run. But in general, I came to agree with the professors. The cattle are better off, except for the part about being slaughtered at the end.

Where You Live and What You Eat

When it comes to human food environments, some are less healthy and more feedlot-like than others. Some places make it easy to eat well, and some people have more resources to resist unhealthy temptations. A study in North Carolina found that Whites were three times as likely as Blacks to have cars, and four times as likely to live in a neighborhood with a supermarket.[10] In low-income communities, it's relatively easy to find liquor stores and fast foods, but produce and whole grains are often out of reach.

In the largely African-American neighborhood of North Vallejo, California, you would have to walk for an hour to find a store selling fresh produce.[11] And I do mean walk, because there are few buses. As one neighborhood activist said, "The types of stores that are here, they're not selling [health] drinks. They're selling pork and grease! That's because there's no transportation, no way out to shop in better stores."

Even if people can access healthy food, they may not be able to afford it. In general, healthy food is more expensive than food that is bad for you. A 1995 British study found that a shopping cart of healthy food costs 51% more than a cart of unhealthy food.[12]

It's very frustrating for people in such situations to hear advice about eating five to nine servings of fruits and vegetables a day. It's simply unavailable or too expensive for some, while others have never been introduced to them.

Power in the form of resources and motivation has a major effect on people's food environment and their ability to cope with it. Some people in North Vallejo have working cars or access to them, others don't. Some may be motivated to walk to better stores; some may be unable, unwilling or afraid to walk that far. Some have more money than others. With money, you can have food delivered; you can buy gas to drive to the next city with a supermarket; you can eat at a decent restaurant. With no money, you may be dependent on government-supplied "welfare food," which is usually high in fats and sugars.[13] Bridging these equality gaps will require social or political approaches. Communities may have to work together to bring healthier food in, grow their own, go en masse to better stores, demand government help to bring markets to their neighborhood, or open their own.

Sugar as an Addictive Drug

Food companies like to say that it's the consumer's fault for eating too much or eating unwisely. They call this "personal responsibility," and accuse food activists like Drs. Brownell and Nestle of promoting a "nanny society," where government protects people from themselves. Why can't we just let people choose what they want?

Drug pushers make the same argument. Pushers don't force anybody to use, and they never address their own personal responsibility for the addictions of their customers. I can imagine the screams of protest of ADM executives reading this, but the analogy is precise. Sugars and other concentrated carbs like HFCS aren't just unhealthy foods. For many, they are addictive drugs.

Addiction counselor and researcher Kathleen Des Maisons, Ph.D., has labeled this addiction "sugar sensitivity."[14] Drs. Emanuel Cheraskin and Marshall Ringsdorf call sugar "the mother of all addictions,"[15] and biochemist Dr. Candace Pert, author of *Molecules of Emotion,* says, "Sugar is a drug, an external substance acting throughout the brain and body."

According to Des Maisons' and others' research, eating sugars or refined baked goods (which break down rapidly into sugar in the blood) raises blood levels of two chemicals: serotonin and beta-endorphin.[16] As blood glucose rises, so do serotonin and beta-endorphin levels.[17] Raising serotonin levels is how drugs like Prozac and Paxil fight depression. Beta-endorphins are natural versions of opiate drugs like morphine and heroin. These chemicals give you a sense of control and calm. They relieve anxiety and physical pain. That's why sugars (and some fats) are called "comfort foods."

Naloxone, a drug that blocks the high from opiates, also blocks the comforting effects of sugar.[18] If a sugar-sensitive person comes across a platter of fresh-baked chocolate chip cookies, they might eat half the plateful. But if they're on Naloxone, — which is usually used to wake people up from heroin overdose — they might eat just one, because they won't get the feel-good effect. If Naloxone can block sensations caused by certain foods, that is a strong indicator of the drug-like action of those foods.

The problem with sugar — and the refined carbohydrates that turn rapidly into sugar — is that the improved mood won't last long. The pancreas will rapidly pump out insulin to handle the sugar, blood glucose level will drop rapidly, and soon the sugar-eater feels worse than before. Meanwhile, they will have added to insulin resistance and stressed their beta cells. And they will gain weight. So sugar sensitivity may be a road that leads from depression and stress to weight and diabetes.

Are You Sugar Sensitive?

Naturally low levels of serotonin and endorphins might be genetic or they might be a result of prenatal or early childhood environments. Whether a person's levels of serotonin and endorphins are low naturally or low because they're under stress, it's natural for them to try to raise those levels with sugar or refined bread, which is basically sugar in another form.[19] Alcohol and cigarettes can also temporarily reduce stress, but don't taste as good and have negative social effects.

People can probably develop sugar-sensitivity at any age. People who live in stressful situations can gradually become more anxious and depressed, another way of saying their serotonin and endorphin levels may decrease. This can also happen to people who, for whatever reason, eat a lot of sugars over a period of time (for example, at college, after a breakup, or during a time of unemployment when money is tight).

Sugar addiction is much like other addictions. Just as muscle cells start resisting insulin when they have too much glucose, brain cells will start to resist serotonin and endorphins when sugar drives those levels too high.[20] This is called "down-regulation" and occurs when the body has too much of a hormone, another chemical messenger or a drug. Some of the receptors for the hormone or drug close down. As time goes on, in order to get the same effect, the body will crave more and more of the drug — in this case sugar — that produces this effect.

The reverse happens when you try to lower your sugar intake. When the body's levels of serotonin and beta-endorphins are low, the brain "up-regulates." Cells become more sensitive to those chemicals. They want to get hold of every molecule of it that they can, so they grow extra receptors to capture those feel-good compounds. They are "primed" to get a hit.

All carbohydrates eventually break down into sugars, but some do so faster than others. Refined carbs, "white things" like French bread or white rice or hamburger buns, break down quickly and reach hungry cells rapidly, perhaps while the bun is still in your hands. Your brain identifies the source of the good feelings and starts screaming for more. If you're sugar sensitive, the more white carbs you eat, the more sweet stuff your brain will crave.

From studying Des Maisons' work, I disagree with diabetes experts who say that people with T2D can eat anything they want, as long as they are careful about amounts. The thinking is that people don't like feeling deprived, so prohibiting sugar completely will backfire. People will resist. This is true, but because of sugar sensitivity and the priming effect, I think people find it very difficult to eat "just a bit" of refined carbs. Not all people with T2D are sugar sensitive, but for many, if they cheat with some French bread at a birthday party, their body will be craving sweets for several days afterward. It's easier to just skip the white things in the first place.

Sugar and Cocaine

Is it fair to be so hard on sugar? After all, it's a natural substance, and the reason it tastes so good is that, in its natural state, it's good for us. In nature, things that are sweet are almost always safe to eat and good sources of energy.

But white sugar and HFCS are not in their natural state. They're like cocaine, which is made from coca leaves that natives of the Andes Mountains (in places like Bolivia and Colombia) have chewed for thousands of years. It keeps them going; it enables them to live well in a harsh environment. But Europeans came and boiled the coca down into a refined paste that makes people feel too good. It makes them crazy; it addicts them.

So now aircraft employed in the "War on Drugs" come and burn down and poison the poor coca plants and the Bolivians, who have done nothing wrong. It's just the ultra-refining of the coca that makes it toxic. Sugar is the same way. Whole grains, fruits, and vegetables are healthy, natural sources of sugar, but refined, processed sweeteners are drugs. Perhaps the American military will start burning down cornfields to control HFCS, but I doubt it.

Diabetes: Day 1

Babies can start becoming hooked on sugar and fat the day they're born.[21] Many studies show that bottle-fed babies are more likely than breast-fed babies to be overweight,[22] and up to 40% more likely to get diabetes.[23] It's possible that formula encourages sugar sensitivity, although other factors are also likely involved. And while some studies indicate a weaker correlation between formula and diabetes, the US Food and Drug Administration is clear that breastfeeding is better for a child's all around health and well being.[24]

But when the US government put out ads to promote breastfeeding, mentioning the diabetes connection, formula manufacturers complained. The American Academy of Pediatrics backed them, and the ads were greatly softened.[6] Meanwhile, the formula ads continue unchecked. So families are still being pushed to start their babies on a road that may lead to diabetes for someone else's profit.

Formula has saved a lot of lives and made life more convenient for millions of families. (It's also killed thousands of babies in poor countries, where they can't get clean water to mix the formula.) But if infant formula pushes kids towards overweight and diabetes, as it appears to from many studies, we should at least know about it.

Nowhere to Run: Toxic Inactivity

For a steer, the worst thing about living in a feedlot isn't all the food. It's not being able to get out on the hills and mooove around. It's the same with human feedlots. Bodies need to move, but our work, hobbies, transportation, entertainment, even our religious worship require sitting. If it weren't for housework, most of us wouldn't move at all! You can eat a tremendous amount and still be healthy if you exercise enough. But when it comes to movement, we live like we're in jail. In fact, most convicts probably get more exercise than the average free-range American.

Movement is the most important part of keeping healthy, especially preventing diabetes. Glucose (sugar) is fuel, and if the muscles aren't moving, they won't need that fuel. Insulin will keep bringing unneeded glucose to the muscle cells, but in self-defense, the cells become resistant to insulin. For most people in modern societies, inactivity is the primary cause of insulin resistance, the core of Type 2 diabetes.

This stationary environment didn't just happen. Like the toxic food environment, it was imposed on us for profit. Starting in the 1940s, automobiles took over the roads, making walking or biking difficult and dangerous. Auto companies even bought up urban transit systems and shut them down.[25,26] Housing started moving farther from cities, jobs and shopping areas. In many places, there are no sidewalks. You can't walk; you are forced to drive.[27]

On a recent trip to Toledo, Ohio, where I was giving some talks, I didn't see one person walking or riding a bike. Two women in a suburb told me that, because streets are so wide and people drive so fast, they actually drive across the street to get lunch every day. And they work for the Diabetes Association! The auto, oil and construction industries have made a lot of money on urban sprawl and automobiles, but they keep people inactive and damage our health and the environment.

The dominance of cars promotes poor health all over the world. A study of eight provinces in China found that people with cars had an 80–100% greater chance of becoming obese than those without them.[28] (In China and some other developing countries, the well-off are sometimes more prone than the poorest to diabetes because of access to cars and American-style food.)

It's not only the car culture that keeps people sedentary. Television and video games have replaced more active forms of entertainment such as sports, and advertising has played a significant role in this. Compare the profit margins. Ten kids can entertain themselves for hours with one relatively cheap basketball. The same kids might need ten video games and the high-priced game-playing machines to keep them entertained. Schools have cut back on Physical Education programs and sports to save money. In fact, schools are often the classic human feedlots, with children expected to sit still for long periods, then turned loose on vending machines or cafeterias stocked with high-calorie foods.

Work as Exercise?

Work used to be highly physical, sometimes to the point of exhaustion. Now work is still exhausting, but for most of us, not physically. We get mentally or emotionally tired, but our bodies don't get to move. Running a crane isn't like nailing up boards, even if it makes you just as worn out at the end of the day. Physical activity used to be built into life; now it requires a conscious effort to go out and do it, every day, in between your other demands.

Voluntary physical activity is more available and attractive to some people than to others. Some people can join a comfortable gym with a wide variety of equipment and programs. Others are limited to taking daily walks through dangerous streets or doing calisthenics in a crowded apartment. Some have enjoyable lives that seem worth putting effort into, and the effort itself might be enjoyable. Others justifiably see exercise as work that they would rather not do, on top of a mountain of other demands and precious little enjoyment. It's often the people with the hardest lives who also have the most barriers to movement.

Today's working environment discourages movement for many people. I visited a noisy recycling plant in Burlingame, California, where the workers spent eight hours standing at a conveyor belt, pulling glass bottles and metal cans off the line and throwing them in bins. Not exactly a well-designed workout! They weren't even provided with step stools they could have used to vary the position of their feet, so most went home with significant back and shoulder pain and major fatigue. No way were many of them going to exercise after a day like that!

Their wages wouldn't have paid for gym membership, so their opportunities might be limited to walking crime-ridden streets with back pain and tired feet. Where would the motivation come from to do something like that?

Breaking Out of the Lot

We have to get off the feedlot; we have to make a run for it. Fortunately, the feedlot is only a metaphor, and movement is almost always possible. Exercise has countless benefits. It makes people feel better, gives them more energy and confidence. For people who want to start getting healthy, coping with diabetes, or losing weight, it's usually better to start with movement than with worrying excessively about food choices. We'll discuss individual and social ways to engage in physical activity in Chapters 6 and 7. But first, there is the medical response to consider. Is American medicine helping the situation or making it worse? Chapter 4 distinguishes the helpful from the harmful when it comes to modern diabetes medicine.

Chapter

4

The Medical System:
Friends and Enemies

*"In most countries, health care is about how to get well.
In the US, it's about how to get paid."*

— ALF ADAMS

W E LIVE IN A TOXIC social environment that gives people T2D and other chronic illnesses. We rely on our medical system to repair the damage the environment creates. But does the system actually help people get better? Sometimes it does, but this chapter shows how, in many places and situations, medicine actually makes things worse.

It's astonishing to think that a two trillion dollar health care system could actually damage health. But by replicating the power relationships that make people sick in the first place, it has done just that. In the typical medical relationship, a patient goes in, gives the doctor control, follows orders, gets better, or dies. This works in acute situations like trauma, pneumonia, or heart attacks. It doesn't work at all in chronic conditions, where self-care is primary.[1] The medical system can damage people with diabetes in at least six ways:

- Making people physician-reliant instead of self-reliant.
- Sabotaging the self-confidence necessary for diabetes management.
- Focusing on drug therapies instead of on healthy living.
- Isolating people as individual patients instead of bringing them together for mutual support.
- Cutting some people off from care completely (especially in the US) and minimizing services for prevention and self-management.
- Giving dietary advice, ordering medications and setting glucose targets that may be quite harmful to some people with diabetes.

Denying Patient Control

Richard Bernstein is one of the heroes (and unique characters) of the diabetes epidemic. In 1969, he was a thirty-five year old engineer, dying slowly of poorly controlled Type 1 diabetes. He had diabetes-related kidney disease, heart disease and circulation problems in his legs. He had frequent attacks of low blood sugar (hypoglycemia) that incapacitated him and made him a terror to be around. "I had three children, the oldest six years old," he remembers, "and with good reason I was certain I wouldn't live to see them grown."[2]

Then he discovered an ad in a lab supply catalog for a newly invented blood sugar meter that would give a reading in one minute from a drop of blood. This meter was being marketed to emergency rooms for use when labs were closed at night. Bernstein was thrilled by the possibility of investigating his own sugar levels, but the manufacturer said they weren't permitted to sell to patients, only to doctors and hospitals.

Fortunately, Bernstein's wife was a psychiatrist with an M.D. He ordered a meter in her name and started attacking his diabetes problems like an engineer, checking his glucose up to eight times a day. He experimented, trying different foods and testing after each one, changing his insulin doses, finding out what kept his sugars close to normal and what made them soar and crash. He found that if he avoided most carbohydrates and gave himself small doses of fast-acting insulin before every meal, his sugar levels improved dramatically. He had energy; he looked good, many of his medical complications disappeared. His cholesterol and other lab test results returned to normal. The hypoglycemic episodes stopped.

Excited and hoping to help others, Bernstein went to his doctor, a leader in diabetes organizations and author of several books on medical management of diabetes. Bernstein encouraged him to make the glucose meters available to all his patients. The doctor replied, "What are you trying to do, put me out of business?"

"Doctors couldn't do much besides test your sugars and order insulin," Bernstein writes in his book, *The Diabetes Solution*. "If patients could test their glucose themselves, why see the doctor?" But self-monitoring is crucial to managing diabetes. Without it, people find it much harder to maintain control of their sugar levels, because they have to guess at how different foods and exercise affect them, instead of knowing the facts. The issue of power in medicine could hardly be drawn more starkly than this.

Undeterred, Bernstein wrote an article on his success in normalizing his sugars and reversing complications, and submitted it to medical journals. They all rejected him. He had his article typeset and printed at his own expense. He gave copies to Charlie Souther, a sales rep at Miles Laboratories, the meter's manufacturer. Bernstein and Souther gave the articles out at conferences and universities but they didn't get far. "The physician resistance was tremendous," says Bernstein. "It was unthinkable that patients be allowed to 'doctor' themselves."

At age 45, Bernstein put himself through medical school, "so they would have to pay attention to me." But it took years of pushing before glucose self-monitoring won widespread medical support. Even now, insurance coverage for testing equipment is limited.

The Struggle for Self-Management

Because diabetes outcomes depend overwhelmingly on people's ability to care for themselves, health professionals should focus on building patients' self-care capacity. Patients should be in control; health practitioners should form strong, supportive relationships with them, coaching them toward self-care success. This approach is often called "Self-Management Support" (SMS).

SMS is available to very few people with diabetes. Instead, professionals frequently damage people's self-confidence by blaming, labeling and threatening, and by dumping large numbers of behavioral prescriptions on people without giving them support. "Just eat according to this meal plan, exercise regularly, take these medications, check your blood sugars, reduce stress and come see me every couple of months, and you'll be okay. Otherwise, you'll go blind or lose your feet." This kind of ordering and threatening is known not to work; most people can't change their behavior that fast, and they quickly become discouraged.[3]

Other times, professionals withhold knowledge from patients, telling them they have "just a touch of sugar," or "borderline diabetes," without giving them diabetes information or helping them to live healthier lives. Professionals need to work with patients as equals and coaches, rather than offering false reassurance or trying to terrorize them into accepting orders from on high.

Studies show that good communication between patients and providers encourages self-care and leads to better outcomes.[4] Because doctors usually have higher status than patients and frequently know little about their patients' personal lives or struggles, good doctor/patient communication is fairly rare. A Belgian study found that poor communication was a major cause of patients' not following treatment plans.[5] "Doctors can't relate to having a chronic medical condition," was a typical patient comment.

Relationships with physicians are especially problematic for people from subordinate ethnic/racial groups, those with a different language or those who are less educated than their physician. Doctor visits can often be a source of extreme stress for people with little power, including overweight people, who are the majority of those with T2D and are often subjected to blame and shame in the doctor's office. As diabetes expert Dr. Roland Hiss puts it, "Patients avoid encounters with their health care providers about their diabetes because the experience is often demeaning and judgmental."[6]

Power relationships are also reinforced and self-care capacity damaged by medical labeling. Psychologist Ellen Langer found that experimental subjects' performance on tasks could be significantly decreased by being labeled (for example as "worker" or "assistant" instead of "executive").[7] Other studies have found that African-American college students did significantly worse on tests when they had to fill in a box marked "race/ethnicity" at the top of the paper.[8] When we think about the labels people with diabetes are given, it's no wonder that they feel unconfident about their ability to succeed at self-care.

Here's a partial list of labels imposed in the medical system:
- Patient: implies a person who waits passively while someone else takes charge. But passivity is exactly what we don't want to encourage.
- Chronic Progressive: you can't get better, you will have to get worse, and there's nothing you can do about it.
- Obese: from the Latin for overeating, as if that were the whole problem. No mention of stress or inactivity.
- Non-compliant: you won't do what we tell you. (This is

now often replaced with "non-adherent," which means the same thing.)
- In denial: if you don't follow our orders, it's because you can't face the truth about your health and your life.

In addition to these medical labels, there are often accompanying social labels, including educational labels ("dropout"), ethnic labels, job category labels, mental health labels ("depressive"), not to mention all the insulting labels mainstream culture pins on overweight people.

Fortunately, some of these damaging medical practices are changing. Self-management support has gained some acceptance (though it is more often talked about than practiced) in chronic illness care. The diabetes establishment has recognized the importance of patient education. A whole profession of Diabetes Educators has grown up, and the idea of patients' responsibility and empowerment has gained momentum, but there is still a long way to go. Medical control and drug therapy still rule. Self-management is the orphan half-sibling, fed when resources are available, after everyone else has eaten.

The Strip Mall of Western Medicine

Most health educators don't take a vow of poverty, though for the compensation they receive, they may as well have. Diabetes educators are crucial actors in supporting self-management. They teach the myriad details of glucose testing, meal planning, medication use, prevention of foot and dental infections, and psychological coping. They help foster the skills and attitudes people need to make behavior changes and stick to them. Their program, usually called Diabetes Self-Management Training (DSMT) can make a critical difference in people's lives and health outcomes.

Though these educators clearly play a significant role in diabetes care, their paychecks don't reflect this. Most insurers pay pathetic amounts for diabetes education. "Medicare pays for ten hours of diabetes education and DSMT the first year," says Virginia Zamudio, past president of the American Association of Diabetes Educators, "and then two hours a year in succeeding years. The benefit is around $18 per 30 minutes. It's good that we have that benefit; we had to have a law passed to get it. But about 67% of the people with diabetes on Medicare don't have access to DSMT."

A lot of diabetes educators who are registered nurses or dietitians can't bill for Medicare services, because they can't get Medicare Provider numbers. Many providers, especially in rural areas, find the process of becoming Medicare-certified to deliver diabetes education onerous and expensive. "The ADA recognition process requires facilities to begin providing education to clients and collecting organizational data and client data for at least 20 participants during a six month period," according to a recent report by researchers in Alabama and South Carolina.[9] "During this time, the facilities must support the education without reimbursement." That's on top of a $1,050 application fee, and Medicare puts various restrictions on which patients are eligible for services, what professional qualifications educators need and where services can be delivered.

Non-Medicare patients seem to have even less access to DSMT. The low reimbursement rates (and complete lack of coverage in many cases) discourage many health care providers from offering diabetes education/SMT at all. Zamudio set up shop three years ago with two nurses and a dietitian, after their hospital laid off the entire diabetes department because it hadn't made a profit.

Many providers are under severe economic pressure and feel they can't offer DSMT at a loss. "There are a lot of people here who would like to do [education]," said one educator, "but it is difficult to convince the administration if the facility will lose money."

Even the current level of funding is under attack from some medical circles. A recent study in the American Journal of Cardiology reported that increased diabetes knowledge did not improve clinical outcomes in T2D. The authors recommended that money for diabetes education be spent on cholesterol-lowering drugs instead.[10] But experts had long known that knowledge itself doesn't make a difference. It's the self-management skills, the behavior change guidance and the support that improves outcomes, as has been shown in numerous studies.[11]

Drugs First, Last and Always

Why has self-management gotten such short shrift? It's partly because of the power relationships in medicine — "We've got the power and you don't" — and partly because of medicine's domination by the pharmaceutical industry. The industry's influence on the practice of Western medicine cannot be over-stated.[12] Drug money pays for professional journals and subsidizes professional conferences. Drug salespeople visit doctors on a regular basis to promote their therapies.

Walk into a diabetes conference exhibit area, and you'll see an acre of exhibits for glucose meters, sugarless foods, literature and all the paraphernalia of the people who call themselves, without a trace of irony, "the diabetes industry." But the drug companies dominate the scene. There is a dancing pancreas promoting one medication, and teddy bears wearing t-shirts emblazoned with another drug's logo. Drinking cups, note-books, even band-aids carry drug company ads. Because drugs are so profitable, drug studies are usually the biggest and best-funded research projects and receive the most attention from the journals and the public.

What's wrong with this? Haven't new medications made huge improvements in people's health and lives? In a few condi-tions, they have. But most oral medications are ineffective in diabetes — exercise beats them by a mile.[12A] These drugs aren't useless; as part of a self-management program focused on physical activity, healthy eating and stress reduction, they can play a useful role.

The problem is not that the oral medications do harm, although some do have serious side effects, including liver and kidney damage. It's not that they cost so much, although they can consume a major chunk of a patient's monthly budget, causing economic stress. The problem is that stress, inactivity and unhealthy eating cause diabetes, and drugs can't help with those. The drugs are a distraction from what would really help: patients' self-care and management of their condition, which health professionals could enable if they weren't so busy pushing drugs. Dr. Jaime Davidson, a leader of the American Association of Clinical Endocrinologists, points out that "diabetes management has actually worsened in the past ten years"[13] in spite of spiraling drug and treatment costs.

Drug use in T2D can easily become totally out of control. Many T2D patients also have high blood pressure, bad cholesterol levels, depression and sometime heart disease and chronic pain. Most doctors treat each symptom separately, and patients usually wind up on seven, ten, even more medications, with or without insulin injections. I met a man in San Diego recently who was on 20 different medications. He had no idea what most of them were for. Taking this many medications almost guarantees damaging side effects. And they don't treat the problem; they don't get people moving. They just pacify the patients and enrich the drug companies.

The Economics of Diabetes

Economics — specifically, who gets paid — influences every aspect of medical care, often in a way that can harm people with diabetes. The complications arising from poorly controlled diabetes make it potentially one of the most expensive medical conditions. Diabetics who don't or can't take good care of themselves tend to run up huge pharmacy bills and to need surgery, frequently multiple surgeries, on their legs or eyes. They may have heart attacks or strokes and wind up needing long-term care and/or a coronary artery bypass or some other vascular surgery. Most expensive of all is kidney failure, requiring dialysis or a transplant (very expensive procedures) to survive.

By keeping blood sugar levels under control, all of this can usually be prevented, as Dr. Bernstein discovered in 1969. Few doctors accepted the importance of blood sugar control, however, until the US government-run Diabetes Control and Complications Trial (DCCT) (1983–1993) demonstrated the importance of control in a group of 1,440 patients with Type 1.[14] Complications were reduced by 50–75% when patients used frequent monitoring, insulin injections, diet and exercise to keep blood sugars down. In 1998, an important English study called the UK Prospective Diabetes Study confirmed the same thing for people with Type 2.[15]

Now everyone agrees that tight glucose control can prevent and sometimes reverse complications. The key to control is good self-management support, helping patients take charge of the day-to-day decisions that influence their sugar levels. So you would think that providers and insurers would be anxious to provide these services, aggressively pushing their diabetic patients into training programs in order to prevent fantastically expensive future health calamities.

You would be wrong, though. Dr. Thomas Bodenheimer, expert on chronic care and author of several articles on health economics,[16] explains why: "Most insurers turn over their enrollees after a few years; people change or lose jobs, employers change health plans, etc. So it isn't worth insurers' while to do interventions that have a return on investment in 10 years. Somebody else will get the benefit of the services they paid for.

Also, for-profit companies need to look good on Wall Street every quarter, so short-term profit is what is important. If they start to pay for self-management support, that will increase expenses and hurt their present-quarter bottom line." A clear summation of why the market and health care don't mix!

Many insurers cut diabetes costs by pushing people with diabetes off their plans entirely. Dr. Bodenheimer says that, "Individual insurance will either exclude people with diabetes or charge such high premiums that people can't afford the plan." It's not much better for employees of small companies. A Georgetown/ADA study found that some insurers increased premiums for an eight-person business by 37.5 percent if one person in the group had diabetes.[17] As a result of such policies, millions of people with T2D have no insurance at all, and millions more lack the means to pay for medicines or self-management support, even if it were available. They won't be covered until they become disabled enough for Medicare or impoverished enough for Medicaid, and even those programs don't give much support to self-management. The result is often more complications, early disability and death and vastly higher expenses.

Perverse Incentives

You may have noted that denying preventive care to people with diabetes makes no economic sense; it greatly increases total system costs. This outcome is an example of what economists call a "perverse incentive." An incentive is perverse when the economics of a situation drive people to do things they know have more long-term costs than benefits.

The American medical system is filled with perverse incentives. For example, new, patented drugs have much higher profit margins than older generic ones. So companies keep coming out with new ones, promoting them to physicians and patients, and the new drugs often wind up replacing the old ones, even if the older drugs are cheaper, safer and just as effective. According to the former editor of the New England Journal of Medicine, Marcia Angell, in 2002, of the 78 drugs approved by the FDA, only 17 contained new active ingredients and only 7 were classified as improvements over their older versions.[12]

Perverse incentives are guaranteed when you have a fractured medical system with thousands of providers and hundreds of payers. What one considers a cost and tries to minimize, another considers income and wants to increase. This kind of thing can suppress self-management support (SMS). SMS may help patients avoid unnecessary hospital admissions, but if a medical clinic has to pay for SMS, but doesn't share in savings from reduced admissions, the clinic won't keep doing it.

Dr. John Abramson, author of *Overdosed America,* sums up the incentives this way: "Drug companies earn higher profits when more people use expensive drugs, not when people achieve better health. Doctors and hospitals are paid more for doing more, largely without regard for evidence of improved health outcomes.... Health care providers that deliver high quality, efficient care are financially penalized for not delivering a higher volume of more intensive services, beneficial or not. [...] American politics, science, and health care have created an imbalance between corporate goals and public interest that has become resistant to correction."[10]

The perverse economics of American health drives health maintenance organizations (HMOs) and insurers to sign up only healthy people. An HMO is called a "capitated" plan, because the provider receives a set amount per patient per year, regardless of what services are provided. So HMOs profit from doing less. HMOs and insurers don't benefit from becoming good providers of chronic illness care, because their success will draw other ill people to their plan. For example, Northern Californian HMO Kaiser Permanente cut their patients' rate of death from heart disease by 15% over eight years, among the best coronary care results in the US. In any other industry, they would have been shouting this success from the rooftops, but Kaiser was very low key about it. As one physician told me, they couldn't afford to have cardiac patients beating down their doors.

Good diabetes care does even worse in the fee-for-service model, where providers profit from doing more, as long as their services are covered by insurance. In the late 90s, four New York City hospitals set up diabetes training centers to help people manage their condition effectively. Although the centers were unqualified clinical successes, three of them closed within seven years because they lost too much money. But more than 100 kidney dialysis centers operate in the city, treating diabetes' most expensive complication, with more opening every year. According to the *New York Times,*[18] providers can "lose money on prevention...or make money on complications" — a truly perverse incentive.

Virtually all other industrialized countries spend far less on health than the US yet get better care and better outcomes.[19] Canada spends about half as much per capita on health care as the US, but has better health outcomes in almost all categories.[20]

It is hard to conceive of a way that the US can make sane, cost-effective, health-promoting choices in this chaotic economic environment. We're moving more and more to market forces, even though the market has been shown completely ineffective in controlling costs or maintaining access when it comes to health.[16] How can the market make rational decisions when the payer (the patient or insurer) is not the primary decision-maker (the physician or health professional)?

The major form of health care competition for HMOs is the fight to sign up healthy patients and get rid of sick ones. Fee-for-service operations compete to provide expensive services, which they are compensated for, while unloading uncompensated ones that often have more value for patients. This competition only adds layers of marketing and administrative costs to an already bloated system. Rational decisions about where to spend health resources require a single-payer plan, so that all costs and benefits come out of the same account.

Single-payer does not, however, necessarily ensure good decisions. National Health Services (NHS) in Canada and elsewhere are under huge financial strain from the growing cost of drugs and chronic illness care. We need an NHS that focuses on wellness and self-management support, as well as strong public health departments to work for healthier environments. Only then will be able to control costs and improve health care.

Medicine as Scam

The medical establishment has two reasonable-sounding arguments for maintaining the focus on drugs and surgery. First, they say that other approaches are not cost effective. They point out that self-management support costs money, which may not be completely compensated by savings in other areas such as reduced hospitalizations or surgeries.

But why should mind/body and social approaches be expected to pay for themselves? Drugs and surgery don't have to be revenue neutral. They cost the system a lot of money, but if they can show some modest clinical benefit, they will be paid for without much question. If drug therapy had to be cost effective, Americans would not be paying half of the world's total drug expenditures — about $200 billion annually out of a worldwide $400 billion.[12]

For my illness, multiple sclerosis, new drugs have been marketed in the last 15 years that cost $1,100–$1,500 per month or even more! They don't cure; they don't even claim to make anyone feel better. They slow down the rate of progression of MS symptoms in some patients by an average of 25–30%, and patients are expected to take them for the rest of their lives. You can argue that these drugs are effective, but cost-effective? And we already know that T2D medications are cost-ineffective compared to exercise, which has proven benefits and is essentially free.

Cost-effectiveness decisions are skewed by the question of who receives the money. In the self-management and social approach to diabetes, mid-level professionals, low-level health workers and patients themselves do most of the work. The high-paid beneficiaries of medical and surgical approaches have no economic reason to support social approaches, and they are calling the shots right now.

Where's the Evidence?

A related deceptive argument is the concept of evidence-based medicine. It sounds good. Relying on the evidence of scientific studies, instead of on the judgment of individual practitioners makes sense. Studying different approaches and disseminating the results to all providers should lead to better quality care for more patients, and sometimes it does.

The problem is that these studies take time and cost money, and the drug companies have more of these resources. They pay for studies at multiple medical centers, enrolling huge numbers of patients. This leads to results with more statistical power. A relatively small benefit can be statistically convincing if the number of subjects is large. So drug use can claim to be evidence-based.

But a study of an SMS approach, say using lay people with diabetes to teach self-management skills to others with T2D, will probably be run on a shoestring. A few do-gooders in the clinic will be putting in volunteer time after their regular shift to construct the study and run it, analyze the results and write it up. The numbers of subjects will usually be much smaller, because you only have so much time, energy and money. The result is a study with less statistical power. Even if the benefits are greater than in the drug trial, they don't look as impressive because of the smaller numbers. The "p-value" (the possibility that the results could have happened by chance) will be higher in a smaller study, and a very low p-value tends to be what people look for in evaluating the significance of a study.[21]

The possibility of procedural weaknesses and mistakes is also much greater in studies of social and mind/body approaches because there's often no paid expert to guide the research. With clinicians instead of experienced researchers running the study, technical mistakes are more likely. It can also be difficult to clearly define and describe exactly what you're doing in a social intervention, a problem drug research doesn't have.

Basing treatment on evidence is a good idea in theory. The American Association of Diabetes Educators has started developing serious evidence on the value of self-management training. They have standardized self-care behavior goals and begun to capture data on the results of different approaches at the local and national level. This effort is being carried out by diabetes educators at the grassroots level but has also been supported by diabetes industry companies Novo Nordisk, Roche, Bayer, Lilly, BD, Lifescan and Ross Abbott. Their work will help to secure funding for self-management support, but for now, medicine is still being steered in the direction of the therapies that are most profitable, because they can afford the biggest studies.

Is There a Cure?

Some people with diabetes believe that medical science is not pursuing a cure because the system makes so much money "managing" diabetes and treating its complications. While there is a bit of truth in that somewhat paranoid economic analysis, it's highly unlikely that any medicine will ever become available to cure T2D, at least, not without causing other problems that could be worse. In my opinion, our glucose metabolism is too deeply ingrained to be safely treated by altering body chemistry with drugs.

There may well be other cures, however. Bariatric surgery (gastro-intestinal bypass operations) seems to have cured a lot of people with T2D. After bariatric surgery, people have to eat very differently than others do — taking much smaller amounts more frequently — and their bodies react differently to food. They absorb food differently because areas that used to absorb food are now cut out of the digestive process. In some, yet unknown way, these changes often bring T2D to a halt.

Serious self-care — lots of exercise, healthy eating and stress reduction — may not completely cure T2D but it certainly improves it substantially. Many advocates also believe that a very low carbohydrate diet is a virtual cure for T2D.[32] This belief is the biggest controversy in diabetes care.

Dietary and Medical Advice Controversies

In the interest of full disclosure, I have to admit that I like and respect the American Diabetes Association (ADA). They do great advocacy, provide services and fund research. They publish some of the best books on self-care and self-management support. I have been paid for speaking at their events, and hope to continue doing so. Keep that in mind as you read the following.

Some of the mainstream advice about diet, medications and glucose control targets may have been influenced by factors other than scientific knowledge, with harmful results for people with diabetes. The diabetes establishment advocates eating 45–65% of calories from carbohydrates, a number significantly higher than the typical American diet (40–45%). Some ADA publications advocate "making starches the star" in diet plans and give advice for increasing starch intake.[22] On the face of it, this seems strange advice. Critics like Dr. Lisa Jovanovic, of California's Sansum Medical Research Institute, point out that people with diabetes (especially Type 1, but to some degree, Type 2 as well) do not have enough effective insulin to handle much carbohydrate. Few disagree. The ADA web page quoted above says, "Your doctor may need to adjust [read: raise] your medications when you eat more carbohydrates." People with diabetes who eat a lot of carbohydrates will tend to have wide swings in their blood sugars, possibly causing damage on both ends, fostering complications.

What is the basis of this high-carb intake advice? When these guidelines emerged, nobody knew for sure what caused diabetes complications. Sugar was suspect, of course, but there were no good human studies on glucose control and complications. (There were animal studies, but they were largely ignored, partly because some experts felt that controlling glucose in humans was too difficult.)

Most people with diabetes die from heart disease or stroke and most of these victims have high cholesterol and triglyceride levels. In line with the accepted nutritional advice of the time, leading diabetes experts recommended low-fat diets to protect people's arteries, but this meant that the lost calories from fat would have to come from elsewhere. Hence the high-carb diet.

Since this advice came out in the mid-80s, the Diabetes Control and Complications Trial (DCCT) and the United Kingdom Prospective Diabetes Study (UKPDS) conclusively showed that diabetes complications are due mostly to poor glucose control. At the same time, a number of studies have shown that high-carb diets may be just as problematic as fat intake in raising blood pressure and triglycerides for many people.[23-26]

ADA spokespeople say they haven't seen strong enough research to cause them to change their recommendations; there are many conflicting studies. There are groups of people, many in the developing world, who have low rates of T2D despite a diet that is relatively high in carbohydrates, and there are studies that show no appreciable advantage to a low-carb approach. Richard Kahn, Chief Scientific and Medical Officer for the American Diabetes Association, says, "We don't have enough data, and it's very difficult to study long-term effects of dietary changes in the real world, where people often don't know exactly what they're eating."

But if it's so hard to perform reliable studies, what is the old advice based on? To the extent that it follows the US Department of Agriculture "food pyramid," it is suspect. The pyramid is determined more by food industry politics than by science, according to such leading nutritional experts as Walter Willett[27] of Harvard University and Marion Nestle[28] of New York University. The committees that develop the pyramid are influenced by food industry sources and normally include many participants with food industry links, who consistently work to emphasize economic considerations over health. And if good studies are so hard to do, how will the ADA's advice every change?

The right diabetes diet may well be a question of individual differences. As Dr. Kahn says, "Diet may need to be individualized when it comes to the impact of diet on blood sugar." Few people with T2D, however, are recommended an individualized diet. Customizing diet would mean people taking charge of their own treatment; checking their own sugars after consuming various foods until they learned how those various foods affect them. Very few practitioners help people with this process. They usually just prescribe a general diet and hope for the best, either because they don't have the time or don't know how to work collaboratively with patients to manage their T2D. Once again, it comes back to a question of who is in control — the doctor or the patient.

Because many people with diabetes end up following generic medical advice and never learn how foods affect their sugar levels, they may be eating much more carbohydrate than is good for them. I interviewed six people for this book whose diabetes had been out of control until reducing their carb intake; they say they are now doing much better on a low-carb diet. Of course, not all carbs are the same. "Brown" and "green" carbs (complex, high fiber carbohydrates such as whole grains, fruits and vegetables,) are more likely good for you than simple carbohydrates (such as breads and sugars). Fats are not all the same, either. Unsaturated fats, such as those from fish and nuts are fine, but saturated (animal) fats may need to be limited. Eating the right type of nutrient may be more important than relative quantities for many people.[29]

Dr. Jovanovic calls the mainstream diabetes diet advice "malpractice."[30] If she's right, it's malpractice on a grand scale. People the world over look to American experts for the best evidence-based recommendations; their advice affects literally millions of people with diabetes. Offering up faulty food advice would place diabetes patients the world over in harm's way. (I'll say more about diet in the Self-care Appendix.)

Saving Beta Cells

Other aspects of modern diabetes care may also harm patients. The most prescribed oral medications are sulfonylureas. These drugs goose the pancreatic beta cells into producing more insulin. Some diabetes experts think these drugs are harmful; that they wear the beta cells out. Robert S. Dinsmoor, a Contributing Editor of *Diabetes Self-Management* magazine, wrote, "Sulfonylureas tend to overwork the pancreas until it eventually "burns out" and is unable to secrete an adequate amount of insulin, so roughly 5% to 10% of people who initially respond to sulfonylurea therapy will subsequently fail each year."[31] Sulfonylurea defenders point out that other studies have found that about the same percentage fail on other types of drugs, so the question is not decided yet.

Dr. Richard Bernstein and others say beta cells can be preserved and even recover considerable lost function by normalizing blood sugars. His treatment involves low-carb eating, exercise, and providing some supplemental insulin. And, like insulin, another class of drug, the thiazolidinediones, can take pressure off the overworked beta cells.

A study in African-Americans in New York found that forty-two percent recovered their glucose-stimulated insulin production (meaning they essentially became non-diabetic, at least temporarily) after only 83 days of near-normal glucose levels. These patients were treated with self-management support; some also received thiazolidinediones. The lead researcher in this study wrote that his study showed, "Therapies directed at promoting beta-cell recovery and preservation are potentially useful approaches to the treatment of Type 2 diabetes mellitus."[32] But most diabetes authorities say nothing about preserving beta cells and continue to prescribe medications that may hasten their demise.

Diabetes doctors and professional organizations often do not advocate the tight blood sugar control that leads to optimal results. Blood sugar control is best monitored by a hemoglobin A1C test, which gives a picture of average sugar level over the previous four–eight weeks. Normal A1C levels of 6% or less would be optimal conditions for prevention of complications, but the ADA's recommended target for diabetics is 7% — even though at this level, people face considerable risk of complications — and most people with T2D run significantly higher than that. There are good reasons for this looser approach — mainly fear of hypoglycemia and patient preference for a less demanding regime. Some patients like the feeling of safety of having slightly elevated sugars; there's less chance of going too low.

But tighter control has been attained by thousands of people and leads to better outcomes and fewer complications. People with an A1C of 7% still face considerable risk of complications. It seems that tight control should certainly be offered as an option. The American Association of Clinical Endocrinologists pushes for a 6.5% norm, and many diabetes educators advocate aiming for 6.0%.

In the New York study of African-Americans cited above, the average patient reached an A1C of 6.2%. These were not specially-motivated self-care zealots; they were people who just happened to be diagnosed during the study. In talking with medical experts for this book, I consistently heard about what people can't do or won't do to modify their behavior and manage their T2D. Some doctors use this argument to explain why they don't push for tighter control, but it's clear to me that lack of support is the much more likely explanation for people's failure to change.

Changing for the Better

Despite the flaws in the system, medical practice is slowly becoming better and more democratic. The ADA has become a leader in supporting self-management research. Some physicians are starting to share power with nurses, dietitians, medical assistants and other providers, and some providers with patients and families. Some systems are moving away from isolating patients and physicians, and are moving toward group practices and group appointments, which are far more effective (see Chapter 7 for a more extensive discussion of this topic).

Leading health reform organizations like the Institute for Healthcare Improvement (IHI) hold trainings and conduct research on involving patients as empowered partners in care. The Institute for Family-Centered Care works tirelessly to involve patients in health care planning processes all over the country. I met some of these patient activists at an IHI meeting in San Diego. They're starting support groups, helping doctors understand patients' needs and teaching self-management from their own experience. We'll see more of the positive side of medicine in coming chapters.

Diabetes educators are changing too. For many years, they were part of the problem, dumping information and behavior change prescriptions on patients without giving them self-management support. But thanks to the groundbreaking work of people like Martha Funnell and Robert Anderson at the University of Michigan and Kate Lorig at Stanford, among others, educators are learning to put patients in charge and effectively support them.

Funnell calls her approach "empowerment,"[33] and it's spreading. She'll tell patients, "My job is to work with you. You're in charge. We're going to work together to come up with something. And if it doesn't work, it doesn't mean you're bad, or I'm bad, it just means we didn't come up with the right plan." Then they try something different.

Empowerment was met with incredulity when Funnell and Anderson started, but it's gaining ground in diabetes education circles and elsewhere. "Twelve years ago, people thought we were crazy," says Funnell. "They truly did. Now it's accepted. I knew empowerment was okay when I heard two old-time endocrinologists give talks, and both said, 'what we have to do is empower patients.'"

When empowerment becomes the basis of medical care, then the medical system will truly be part of the solution. Changing medicine will go together with changing social inequality and the harmful environments of food, inactivity and stress. Health care providers and systems will be leading participants in the movement that is described in detail in Part II.

Part II — Health as a Movement

O N A CHILLY NOVEMBER evening in Oakland, about 120 African-American women, men, and youth are gathered in a small meeting hall. Some have diabetes; some do not. One after another, they report on what they have done to better care for themselves in the last three months, and how they have helped each other do so. They describe exciting plans for future health work — speaking at their churches about nutrition, organizing walking clubs in their neighborhoods, and always, always, committing to self-care. This meeting is a graduation ceremony for the "Health Conductors." Started by local African-American community leaders and consciously modeled on the Underground Railroad, which led Blacks out of slavery, they are determined to lead their people to better health. They are some of the leading lights in the new movement I will call, for now, Diabetes Wellness.

At about the same time, in San Diego, another part of the movement is meeting. Twenty teams of health providers from around the country have come to teach each other "Self-management Support" or SMS. SMS means empowering patients and families and supporting them to meet their goals. It means fully using resources: educators, nurses, medical assistants, community workers, as well as physicians, and putting them at patients' disposal. It is a step away from the medical dominance that is so destructive of healthy living.

And in the streets of Santa Ana, the dedicated organizers of Latino Health Access (LHA) are holding classes, linking people in support groups, creating places for people to exercise and bringing in healthy food. Communities across the country and around the world are doing likewise. They fight City Hall; they get some of their members into office. These three forces: individuals, health care systems, and communities, are the building blocks of the Diabetes Wellness movement. If they connect with other social movements, if they move to challenge and change the unjust and unhealthy social environment, and if they get some support from governments, they might succeed in stopping the diabetes epidemic.

Why We Need a Movement

Part I showed that diabetes (and many other chronic diseases) are socially created. The environment is toxic, and people with less personal or social power get sick because they can't defend themselves. Health can be socially created, too. We can change the toxic environment and create social structures that enable and promote self-care. But when so many social conditions need such significant change, and when these conditions are strongly defended by people who are making billions of dollars from them, we need a social approach to change them. We need a movement.

When I started researching this book, I didn't know that such a movement is already under way. I thought it was a dream, but it's happening all across America and the world. It's not a movement in the sense of big political organizations with 12-point programs holding rallies for the TV cameras. Most people in the movement don't know they're in it or know about other forces on their side. That's what the rest of this book is about.

In addition to patients, their families and the health care providers, the Diabetes Wellness movement involves community groups not normally associated with health or politics. Much of the organizing and action takes place in churches and centers of spiritual life, and people of faith are major participants. Schools are central to the wellness movement, and much of the strength and motivation comes from youth. Politicians play important roles in this movement too, but the leadership naturally comes from the people most affected. In many cases, the health activists and workers themselves become leaders, not just about health issues, but also in dealing with the social conditions that impact people's lives.

A Different Kind of Movement

Dr. Melanie Tervalon, a Health Conductors leader, says this movement is unique, as it starts with self-care. "Unlike many organizing activities that have happened in our community, where it's about everybody else, this is about you taking responsibility for your health every day, so that you are an example, and so that when someone asks you a question about what to do, you don't sound like you're lying."

The people in this movement recognize that self-care has a social context. The support of other people is crucial to regaining health, so the movement consciously sets out to strengthen families and communities. America Bracho, a Venezuelan doctor and community leader in Southern California, says, "As Latinos, we are constantly made aware of the many things we don't do, of all that is wrong. But as health workers, we identify and build on the community's assets. We make each other stronger."

This commitment to each other is at the core of the movement. "We want our community to get well," says Dr. Tervalon. "We're willing to do what's necessary for that to happen."

Where Is This Movement Going?

Stopping the diabetes epidemic and moving towards wellness is a daunting project. There's a tremendous amount of work to be done and a variety of approaches to try. Key approaches include supporting children and families to reduce stress and get children off to a healthy start, increasing physical activity and eliminating barriers to activity, and changing food norms and environments. Diabetes wellness involves basic changes to the health care system, a movement towards a system that focuses on wellness, self-management and prevention for everyone, instead of exotic and expensive therapies for the few.

These are some of the issues the movement is working on, but even bigger challenges are ahead — increasing equality, reducing and managing the stress inequality causes, creating a society where everyone knows they are valued and cared for. No one thinks this will be easy; it will involve profound social change. As you'll see in the coming chapters, small farmers and businesses, environmentalists, labor unions, health workers and social justice advocates are all contributing. But they can't do it alone. Your contribution is needed, too.

Chapter 5

From Shame to Strength

*"I think I got diabetes because I can't control my weight.
I'm frustrated because I don't have the self-control to watch
my diet like I should. I think I potentially have a lot of control,
but I'm not taking that control. And that's the guilt.
It's a vicious cycle."*

— MARIO, AGE 60, STOCKTON, CALIFORNIA

MANY DIABETICS, LIKE MARIO, blame themselves for having diabetes or pre-diabetic weight conditions. Why wouldn't they? As we've seen, doctors and other authorities have been blaming them — their behavior, their genes, or some combination of the two — for years. Health "experts" call T2D a "lifestyle disease," implying that people choose it for themselves. Heavy people are called "obese," which comes from the Latin for "over-eating," as if that were the sole cause of the problem.

But we know that stress, physical inactivity and a toxic food environment cause overweight and T2D in people who lack the social, personal or genetic power to resist. Undeserved blame increases the powerlessness that causes diabetes in the first place. Feeling guilty or ashamed, weak or inadequate heightens stress and can prevent people from making desirable changes.

Shame can be crippling in another crucial way. It keeps people from sharing and from talking to each other about their problems. As a result, people with health problems like T2D are left to deal with them on their own, which is a recipe for failure. Worse still, the social forces that cause illness do not get addressed. Society never realizes who is really to blame, so things continue on as they have been, destroying the health of children and of generations to come.

Stopping the diabetes epidemic requires a movement, and shame and guilt stop people from joining it. Let's look at where the guilt and blame come from, why we have to overcome them, and how that can be done.

A Culture of Blame

Why are people with T2D blamed for it? Much of it has to do with weight. In this society, being overweight equals being bad.[1] Obesity expert Kelly Brownell says, "[Being overweight] has been considered a consequence of weak discipline, laziness, psychological dysfunction or personal failings." If you're heavy, you're weak; you're not worthy of respect or love. You don't know enough, care enough or have enough willpower to live a healthy life.

It's not just weight. This culture likes to blame people for their health problems, because it takes the focus off unhealthy social conditions, and because it makes healthy people feel it can't happen to them.

It's interesting how our society treats people with illness differently, depending on the currently accepted scientific explanation of the illness and on the social groups who have it. With MS, for example, there is no known cause, and nobody blames me for it. On the contrary, when I go out in public with my walker or my cane, people tell me how courageous and inspiring I am. But people with T2D — a chronic condition just like MS — get blamed, and they may be shamed, pitied, or scorned.

They may absorb some of these attitudes from society or from their doctors. It would be hard not to, but these attitudes aren't fair. They aren't based on fact, and they're not helpful.

When people aren't blamed as individuals for their health problems, their culture or ethnicity often gets blamed. "It's the food," people will say, the tamales, the soul food, the fry bread, spaghetti or whatever it is your people eat. "It's our genes." Why else would so many of us be sick or overweight? "Our people were conquered so we must be weak. There's so much crime and violence, so few jobs. What's wrong with us?" All of these arguments move the blame from the individual to the group level, but they're still wrong and they're still harmful.

Feeling guilty or powerless cripples people physically and emotionally. People with T2D are (at least) twice as likely as others to be depressed.[2] A study conducted at Veterans Administration hospitals in the U.S. found that over 60% of patients with T2D reported chronic pain[3] [as compared to 18–22% in the general population[4]]. The usual explanation for these findings is that diabetes is painful and depressing, but this misses the point. More often, the powerlessness people feel is contributing to the depression, the pain, and the diabetes.

Native American researcher Ane McDonald says, "Indians are tired of being blamed for everything." I'm sure African-Americans and other people of color are too, as is anybody else (such as most overweight people) who has been consistently blamed for being the way they are. Feelings of shame and failure have direct health effects through the chemistry of the stress response, and indirect effects through behavior. Gaining a more positive sense of self can heal, as the following study shows.

Trauma and Pride

In a 1995 study[5] of Pima with diabetes (one of the few useful ones), participants were randomized to two groups. One group, called Pima Action, received a structured program of exercise and help with diabetes self-management skills. The other group, called Pima Pride, met with tribal elders and learned about their culture and history (in other words, got a more positive sense of themselves).

The experimenters thought of Pima Pride as sort of a control group to the real intervention, the exercise program. They were shocked when, after 18 months, the Pima Pride group had better results in every outcome — weight, blood sugar control, waist size. A third group of people who declined to participate became the controls. Their outcomes were worse than either of the participating groups, showing that exercise did help. But Pride — which built self-confidence and self-esteem — was significantly better.

Do you see how this experiment could apply to anyone with a chronic illness such as T2D? Few of us are living through an ongoing genocide. But most people have suffered some kind of trauma or faced social or economic stresses that damage their bodies. All of us are living in toxic environments. All of us struggle with taking care of ourselves. And the struggle is much harder if we don't feel we can do it, or don't believe we're worth the effort. Sense of self directly affects people's self-care behaviors and health status.

Note that the more positive self-concept induced by Pima Pride was not based on individual personal growth, but on sharing the community's story. Bookstore shelves across America are filled with individual approaches to building self-confidence and self-esteem. These can help some people, but raising a group's concept of themselves is a way of helping everyone in the group.

Communities against Shame

Other Native American communities have had success with such cultural approaches to building individual and group strength. In a Yup'ik town in coastal Alaska, when some girls were having emotional and behavioral problems — including planning group suicide — tribal elders and mental health workers got the families into a tribal dancing program.[6]

"When a person comes into dance, you are creating a setting that is fun," according to Native psychologists writing in the Healthy Alaska 2010 handbook. "They learn traditional stories as they are learning Eskimo dance. And when you make a mistake, everybody bursts out laughing, including you. So you learn that everybody makes mistakes, and even mistakes can be fun sometimes." There is nothing to be ashamed of.

Other Alaskan tribes have brought back traditional Native games to connect people to their culture while promoting exercise, but traditional practices don't necessarily have to involve physical activity to be helpful. The Yup'ik use steam baths as a venue for sharing stories and emotions and for solving problems. Sweat lodges serve this purpose in many Indian communities, not just on the reservations. Ane McDonald and her partner Francisco run sweat lodges for urban Indians living in the area of Sacramento, California.

Similar problems and approaches apply in African-American communities. Researcher Elaine Peacock reports the words of one pastor in a community wracked with diabetes, who said, "African-American life is devalued in this nation, and this devaluation feeds into people not caring for themselves. We must rebuild our communities and help our people accept themselves."

Confusing Strength with Power

These self-concept issues affect more than just oppressed communities. An individual of any background can have problems with self-esteem and self-confidence. People feel guilty and ashamed and powerless over their lives, not only their health. Maybe everyone you see on TV is richer than you — it must be your fault. Maybe you're lonely and everybody else seems to have friends — you must not be worthy. Or maybe you don't think you live up to your parents' standards and hopes, or don't feel you're doing a good enough job taking care of your family. Maybe you feel guilty for dropping out of college. Maybe you're unemployed. Most people in your community might be unemployed too, but you still blame yourself.

According to Dr. Gabor Maté, author of *When the Body Says No,* much of the shame arises because people confuse strength with power and powerlessness with weakness. Cheryl Sampson, a Community Wellness Advocate (CWA) in Southeast Alaska's Native villages told me, "Diabetes is a sign of weakness, and we don't like weakness." But in some Native American, Pacific Islander and African-American communities, 60% of adults have T2D! This cannot be a problem of personal weakness. It's a problem of social power. In fact, surviving in these oppressed communities requires tremendous strength, and such people should be greatly admired. Yet people of all races and ethnicities continue to blame themselves and never talk about diabetes.

People who are willing to come out and talk about problems like diabetes are the truly strong ones. They can help entire families and communities move forward and gain control of their lives. So often people suffer alone with their health problems, but they don't need to. We can reach out to each other, and those who do are heroes.

Consciousness Raising

In the women's liberation movement, they called this approach "consciousness raising." Women would meet in organized or informal groups of 5–20 to talk about their experiences and the social realities that caused them. They built a huge movement and made a lot of important changes (for example, changing wife abuse and child abuse from accepted normal behavior to a crime.) Women stopped blaming themselves; they fought back, and society changed for the better.[7]

We could use a movement like that for diabetes. Using another example of an oppressed group, Elaine Peacock says, "Community interventions must encompass a consciousness-raising element that causes African-Americans (and others) to respond to conditions of poor health and premature death with an outrage similar to that aroused by racial discrimination and other acts of social injustice."

What about people with T2D who aren't part of an oppressed or disempowered community? If you've read this far, you know that social conditions and power relations play a big part in most cases of diabetes in any community. People may benefit from using support groups or some such gathering for consciousness-raising about the issues that affect them.

Most consciousness-raising starts with knowledge. What social forces are causing our problems? Where do our harmful behaviors come from, why do we continue them, and how can we change them? Where are potential sources of help, and what obstacles are in the way? The idea isn't to find someone else to blame so you can let yourself off the hook. The point is to understand that it's not your fault so you can take the steps you need to get better and maybe help others to do so as well.

The process varies for different groups, as the environment of a Pacific Islander, for example, is different from that of a military veteran, or a woman who has been abused or an inner-city African-American. But the concept is applicable for everyone.

Barriers to Consciousness

There are two main reasons why the truth about diabetes remains hidden. The first we've already covered — the torrent of wrong, blame-the-victim type information washing through our culture. That can only be countered by educating ourselves and each other. The other significant barrier is the pain and fear

The truth can be particularly painful when the stories are traumatic. Cheryl Sampson of central Alaska's Inupak nation, says her people's trauma can be overwhelming for the wellness workers. "In the small rural communities, the unemployment rate is really high — 65, 75, even 85%. We're dealing with the men who are not able to take care of their children, and the problems that are associated with that. The financial worries, the trauma that we are in as indigenous people, the death of our culture, the rapid changes, all these social issues, personal issues, the hurt and the pain."

Sampson (whose traditional name is Agnaqin) is eloquent about her people's pain and its origins. "There is pressure from the state and the federal government to become more Western. The Western society needs oil. The Western society needs coal, needs natural resources. And guess where it's at? It's on our land. So the pressure is great to conform because the Western society needs those natural resources. They're the majority, we're the minority. So it's an out of control situation. Feelings of hopelessness and despair over the loss of your culture, and greater trauma and despair over our babies, over our children, that they are going to live in the current mess that we're in. And that is the greatest trauma — that our children will be in this muck and this mire that we're currently in. I believe that is at the root of all the cancer, the diabetes, the alcoholism, the heart disease, the strokes, these are all symptoms of that trauma. People that smoke, that's self-medication. People that have diabetes because of the sugar and the junk that they eat, they're self-medicating. People that are drinking are self-medicating."

Agnaqin is a brave and wise woman. She says she will do what it takes — cry, work out, spend a week in the forest to help her deal with the pain, but most of her people aren't doing that. Perhaps they can't. I asked her if it would help people to talk about the trauma and acknowledge the pain. I didn't like her answer, but I have since heard similar things from activists in other states, so this is not just an Alaska problem. This is what she had to say:

"There's too much hurt and too much emotion, so we just suppress it. I think if we create a safe environment and say, it's okay to have these hurts, it's okay that we're impacted by suicides. 'We're ashamed, but we can acknowledge that.' I think if we created that safe environment, that tremendous healing would take place. And this can only be done at the local level. There's no other way for change in a community except from within, and that's not going to happen until we're ready. And a lot of communities are not ready. It's simply too overwhelming. When we're ready, I hope I'm there."

Perhaps mental health professionals working closely with First Nations people will come up with ways to make this pain bearable so that people can raise consciousness, grieve, come together and heal. I have heard some suggestions. But what would really help is if large numbers of outside people came to their aid politically and enabled them to reclaim their self-determination. I hope the Diabetes Wellness movement and others take on these issues.

From Weight to Wellness

The first five chapters of this book could act as basic diabetes consciousness-raising for anyone, but some will want a deeper understanding. As an example, I'll go into some depth on the subject of overweight, which is often wrongly thought of as being identical to T2D, and always blamed on the heavy person. As the term "obesity" shows, overeating gets all the blame. Well, what really causes overweight? We saw in Chapter 2 that stress is a major factor, and even when it comes to behavior, physical activity is more important than eating. Stress puts more sugar into the bloodstream, where it largely gets converted to abdominal fat if not burned up with vigorous activity.

And what is the relationship between weight and T2D?

It's true that excess weight (especially abdominal fat) is associated with T2D, and that losing weight often makes it better.[8] But that doesn't mean overweight causes diabetes. Most overweight people do not have T2D. Quite possibly, some underlying factors, including genetic variation, stress, and inactivity are responsible for both the weight and the diabetes.

It's interesting to note that liposuction, a surgical procedure that drains fat from the body through a tube, does not seem to affect blood sugar levels much.[9] But bariatric surgery, operations in which the stomach and intestine are restructured to reduce the space available for digesting and absorbing food, sometimes cures diabetes immediately, *even before weight loss occurs*. The changes in digestion, absorption and eating that result from bariatric surgery seem to bring sugars to normal levels.[10] (Since bariatric surgery is so new, we don't yet know how long-lasting these changes will be.)

In other words, fat itself may not be as damaging to health as the behaviors, conditions and stresses that tend to make you fat. These are what need to change. Heavy people who get themselves fit, as shown by exercise tolerance and normal sugar, cholesterol and blood pressure levels, have little more health risk than lighter people.[11] But the social stress of being fat and of the constant struggle to be thin may add significantly to overall stress and contribute to T2D.

For overweight people, weight loss is desirable, this is clear. It takes pressure off the knees and hips, making it easier to be physically active. It often improves blood sugar control and cholesterol profiles,[12] and in general, makes it easier to stay healthy. Still, society's negative attitudes toward overweight are far stronger than health concerns should dictate.

Prejudice and Power

Most social attitudes against weight have nothing to do with health. They're about money. It used to be that only the rich could afford enough food to be heavy. Fat was associated with wealth, so fat was considered attractive. (This is still the case in many traditional cultures today.) Now, when calorie-rich foods are easy to get, thinness is associated with wealth, fat is considered ugly, and the conventional model of beauty is way too thin to be healthy.[13]

The same pattern has emerged with skin tone, among Caucasians and Asians at least. A century or two ago, only rich people could afford to stay inside. Everyone else was out in the fields working. So the whiter you were, the prettier (i.e., wealthier) you were considered.[14] To be called "white as bone china" was a compliment. In the West, the fact that darker-skinned people were conquered and colonized meant that darker skin was associated with less power and was therefore less attractive. Now that most people work indoors, and only wealthier people can afford to travel to warmer climates or idle out of doors, having a dark, rich, tan is considered attractive and healthy (even if it risks skin cancer).

Desiring the physical traits associated with wealth makes sense, as wealth equals the ability to provide for your offspring, an important consideration when choosing a potential mate. But valuing thinness has resulted in devaluing and shaming people who are heavy, in the guise of concern for their health.

The Healing Power of Mercy

Because T2D is a disease of powerlessness, it almost always comes with myriad other life and health problems. By addressing the undeserved blame and shame that disempowered people live with, they can build their self-confidence and make profound changes. They can heal.

As Native diabetes therapist Regina Whitewolf says, "If we could get together and see that we're all in this crisis together, and it's not our fault, we could start to become better people, to treat each other better."

We need this change to happen, because currently there is little mercy for people with T2D and other conditions they have "brought on themselves."

We need for people to be merciful to themselves and each other, and sharing experiences in a group is a valuable tool for fostering those attitudes. Simply getting together to bitch and complain doesn't do much good — there has to be a context of doing something about it, of getting active. This can include self-care, like exercise and cooking programs. It can also mean working on survival issues like community safety, jobs, and school performance, or on changing the community environment. We'll see a lot of these approaches in Chapter 8.

As people's self-concept improves, so does their motivation and ability to care for themselves. The reverse is also true: succeeding at self-care gives people a much stronger sense of themselves and their own capabilities. But there are obstacles to self-care. Chapter 6 will look at what these are and at how people can succeed at it despite the challenges.

Chapter

6

Self-Care as a Political Act

DIABETES EDUCATORS SAY THAT 90% of diabetes care is self-care.[1] Physical movement, healthy eating, self-monitoring and relaxation are far more important than anything the medical profession can do for diabetes (or for most other chronic conditions). But self-care has a social context, and in this society, that context is mostly negative.

Self-care is not something people see on TV or learn in school. Most people have few role models for it, since most parents are too busy and stressed to give their bodies any attention. In fact, self-care goes against everything the dominant culture believes our lives are about and our bodies are for, namely to produce and consume. Occasionally we can help others or enjoy living, but mostly, time not spent productively is time wasted.

We even learn a story about this as kids, the parable of the ant and the grasshopper. The ant worked and slaved all through the year, while the grasshopper goofed off. As a result, the ant had plenty to eat in the winter, while the grasshopper starved. But that ant probably had chronic back pain and high blood pressure at the very least. They never tell you that part, because some elements of our society want us to endorse the ant's work ethic.

So it's not surprising that we take our bodies — the most precious gifts we will ever be given, and the most valuable assets we will ever have — for granted. We treat them like used cars: we drive them to do all our work without putting much effort back into them. And when they break down, we take them to a mechanic (with a medical degree) and say, "Fix this."

With a chronic illness like diabetes, however, you discover they can't fix you. All of a sudden your life is supposed to revolve around self-care. You're supposed to do it 24/7. But you're on your own with it; as we've seen, society is not set up for healthy living, and most people get little self-care support. Families may not want to start eating healthier. Jobs may enforce sitting or standing all day, wearing you out without allowing any exercise. Employers may not let workers test their blood sugar or take the breaks they need. (It may not be safe to let the boss know you have diabetes at all. They might find ways to make your life miserable or let you go.) Wherever we are, we're surrounded by toxic food. Stressors are everywhere, and eating easily accessible but unhealthy comfort food is often the easiest way to deal with them.

Taking the path of least resistance, eating and living as society and media urge you to do, gives people diabetes and other chronic illness. We can sum up the core of self-care in two words: Get active! If you remain passive, the environment will roll you in sugar, fry you in oil, and have you for lunch. So we need to approach self-care with a fighting spirit. We need to claim the right to care for ourselves. Self-care can be a political act, an act of rebellion that says we are worth taking care of, that our lives have value, even if society seems to deny it.

Power and Self-Care

Taking a political approach to self-care means addressing the issues of power that affect one's health. To eat right when surrounded by toxic food, to move one's body off the couch, to relax in an environment full of stresses and dangers — these things involve taking power over one's life. So does strengthening a family or community when the culture pushes isolation and individualism.

Self-care success starts with physical activity, and the more of it the better. It also means people making their own decisions about what's important and what's unnecessary. It means you decide what's good for you to eat rather than reaching for what's at hand or what the TV is pushing. It means paying attention to your body when society treats it as only a means of production or a source of shame.

For most people, self-care won't suffice on its own to handle diabetes, but without it, nothing else will work. Self-care can also be a turning point that makes people more effective in their families and communities. It makes them assertive; it makes them strong. They may become catalysts that help others value themselves, who help whole communities treat themselves better and get well. And that kind of change can prevent not only diabetes, but many other problems, too.

The Power to Change

Self-care requires both personal and social power. Sources of personal power include external resources: money, social status, education and living in a good neighborhood. Internal resources are also crucial: self-confidence, emotional security, knowledge, positive reasons to live and an assertive fighting spirit. (Social power is just as important and is addressed in the following chapter.)

The one indispensable thing people need for self-care is a willingness to change. Change requires four things: confidence (the belief that you can do it), hope (the belief that change will do some good), valuing yourself (the belief that you and your body are worth some effort) and support. Let's first look at self-confidence.[2]

Albert Bandura, a great social psychologist from Stanford University, developed the concept of self-efficacy (SE), which is self-confidence applied to a particular area of life. SE is the belief that you can do the things you set out to do and is the best predictor of whether you will succeed. "People tend to try activities they believe they can accomplish," says Bandura, "and avoid activities where they feel less confident."

Most professionals treat SE as a psychological construct, something inside an individual's brain or personality, but that is not accurate. The same confusion dogs other related constructs such as "locus of control"[3] and "stages of change."[4] Locus of control (LOC) refers to who you think controls what happens to you, whether it's you or outside forces. Generally, an "internal locus of control" is thought to promote behavior change and better health, and an external locus promotes fatalism and inhibits change. "Stages of change" refers to the priority a person gives a behavior change like stopping smoking or beginning to exercise. In these concepts, health professionals should use counseling and teaching techniques to help people move to a more internal LOC or a higher readiness to change.

But if you think about it a moment, you see that these are not primarily psychological factors at all. They mostly reflect life circumstances and histories. If you have never had the power to make much of anything happen, what will that do to your SE? If you haven't had much control in your life, where will your locus of control be? If you believe you have no control over your body because of early abuse or neglect, why would you think you could control your health, your eating or your exercise behaviors? If you are worried about losing your job, paying your rent, or taking care of a zillion other people, how high a priority would you give diabetes management? By ignoring these factors, professionals can inadvertently cause a lot of frustration and add to a patient's sense of failure.

The great breakthrough of Bandura and other SE theorists has been breaking self-confidence down into specific areas and developing strategies for building SE around particular activities. And SE often generalizes to other activities,[5] so people wind up feeling more powerful and more in control of their lives. In an early study of people with snake phobia, Bandura found that, in conquering their fear of snakes (through a program of progressively greater exposure), people gained the confidence to try a number of things they had been scared of before, such as public speaking. People who increased their SE around maintaining an exercise program might do things like get their high school diploma or cut back on their drinking.

Building Self-Efficacy

This is incredibly powerful stuff. Another Stanford researcher, health educator Kate Lorig, RN, DPH, started the Arthritis Self-Management Program, a six week class/support group run by laypeople with arthritis.[6] Participants reported less pain, more ability to carry out their daily lives and less need for medication or doctor visits. But what was causing the benefit? Was it the knowledge students learned, the exercises they did, the relaxation techniques?

When Lorig probed this further, the answer was none of the above. It turned out that people whose self-efficacy scores had increased the most were the ones who benefited, whether they practiced the new behaviors or not.[2] They felt they had more control, which reduced their stress, and they got better. Lorig's program is now given around the world and used for many other conditions, including diabetes.

Lorig and Bandura agree that a key to the self-management program's success has been the use of lay leaders instead of health professionals. One reason is that "vicarious accomplishment" is one of the best ways to build self-efficacy. When people see others like them having success with a behavior or a program, they tend to believe they can do it too.[7]

Lorig has fought for decades to get the lay leaders accepted by the medical profession. Many doctors and professional educators have been extremely reluctant to give up their teacher status or to believe that lay people can be effective educators. What do they know, anyway? All they have is their years of experience and accumulated knowledge. Where are the Ph.D.s and M.D. degrees?

But Lorig believes in people power. She kept saying, "Professionals are experts on an illness, and patients are experts on their lives," and the two groups need to respect each other's expertise. This theory is gaining acceptance in the arthritis world, but only very gradually in diabetes. A small minority of people with diabetes have access to self-management programs. (Many programs that are called "self-management programs" wouldn't meet Lorig and Bandura's criteria. They lack the crucial focus on building self-efficacy.)

Experiencing Success

An even better way to build SE is by actually accomplishing a goal. Most people give up on a behavior change when they feel they are failing. Let's say, for instance, that John agrees with his doctor that he needs to exercise. The doctor tells John he should walk an hour every evening after dinner, and John agrees. But his favorite show comes on after dinner, he needs to help the kids with their homework, the neighborhood isn't safe and his feet are hurting. He only walks two days out of the week, he feels like a failure and his health providers call him "noncompliant" (medicalese for "disobeys our orders"). His SE around exercise will be very low, and it may be years before he tries it again.

What would be an SE-based way of approaching this problem? Someone from Dr. Lorig's program would probably ask the patient how he wanted to exercise, what he wanted to do, maybe give him a menu of activity choices. The best changes are things that people *want* to do, not something somebody else tells them to do. Most people resist being ordered around, and the key to building "internal locus of control" is to give them more control.

But how do you know they'll actually do what they set out to? In the self-management programs, people decide for themselves how many times they'll do something and how much of it they'll do. They determine their "confidence level." On a scale of 1–10, how confident are they of completing their self-made assignment? Experience shows that the confidence level has to be at least 7; otherwise the change won't get done. The important thing is to succeed. It's better to say you'll walk three days this week and actually do it, than to say you'll walk five and do four. The first way builds SE and paves the way for more changes. The second way makes you want to give up.

Other ways to build SE include positive feedback (like keeping a log sheet or noticing blood sugar readings decreasing) and persuasion (remembering past successes and reframing past experiences to highlight the successful elements). Knowledge also helps build confidence.

A higher SE level sometimes spreads to other areas of a person's life and sometimes doesn't. One key factor to transferring it seems be similarity. SE spreads most easily to behaviors similar to the ones you have already mastered.[8] For example, if a person learns to stick to a daily exercise program (a "self-regulatory" skill in psychological jargon), she may feel confident about going back to school or getting a job, where self-regulation is required. If someone learns to speak up to his doctor about medications, he might speak up to a politician or developer who has an influence over his community, or challenge a convenience store owner to put some healthy food at the front of the store instead of the candy and soda pop.

"You Have to Love Yourself"

Self-confidence is a big part of personal power, but people also need to believe that they are worth taking care of, that their bodies' needs are as important as their other responsibilities. I heard a striking statement of this truth when I interviewed James Ratliff, an African-American sales consultant in Pleasanton, California. He was diagnosed with T2D at age 46. He had a demanding job and a growing family, but he had one key asset: he believed in himself.

"At that time," he told me, "I was maybe 30 or 40 pounds overweight. So I changed my diet to eliminate sugar completely, and not eat a lot of carbohydrates. They had this little gym where I lived, and I started getting up at 5 o'clock every morning to work out. Now my sugars are pretty normal."

Is it really as simple as that? I couldn't believe it. I asked Mr. Ratliff how he was able to quickly make such changes, when many other people struggle their whole lives and never get there. I will never forget his answer: "I love myself," he said. "I think that's the best thing I can do. Once you love yourself, then you're going to take every resource possible to extend your life. That's not being selfish. Sometimes you have to do things for yourself before you can do things for anybody else. If I don't care about myself, how can I care about anybody else? These things are important to understand, that if you want to continue to stay on this planet and breathe this air, that you have to love yourself."

I'm not sure how many people, with or without diabetes (especially members of ethnic groups who are discriminated against or heavy people in fat-phobic America) could say that. How do people love themselves when society does not seem to love them? When all around them is physical evidence that nobody outside their community cares? Or when a person feels unlovable because of absent or damaged parents, a history of trauma, or because their life doesn't measure up to the images they see on TV or to their own expectations.

But if you don't love yourself, why and how are you going to succeed at diabetes self-care? Why watch your carbs or check your blood sugar or get up in the morning to exercise like James Ratliff does? And if you don't love yourself, why expect your children to love themselves, or others in your community to treat each other well? These issues can determine quality of life and health generation after generation. So what do we do?

Self-Love, Family and Community

Self-love is not selfish. It's highly contagious, which is great news because there are so many people who desperately need it. James Ratliff has been able to inspire many friends and neighbors to eat well and exercise, and has gotten his children to live healthier lives than most kids. But it doesn't stop there. His son can pack water in his lunch instead of soda, and can tell his friends, "That cola stuff made my Dad sick. I don't want that for me, and you shouldn't either."

Self-love starts in early childhood. Mr. Ratliff thinks he got it from his mother. Parents are best placed to build children's sense of self, but they are often too stressed to do it. One of the most important things we can do as a society or community to improve health is to support parents and young children.

Social support systems — anything from family and friends and community to large-scale programs — can strengthen people's sense of self. Professionals such as therapists or clergy members can help people reframe their stories to feel more optimistic and less judgmental.[9] The next chapter shows how communities can consciously build self-confidence and self-love.

No More Nice Girl!

Canadian doctor Gabor Maté's excellent book, *When The Body Says No: The Cost of Hidden Stress,*[10] persuasively presents the idea that if you are unable to say "No," your body will say it for you, by getting sick or even dying. Some people are in a better position to say no than others. Obviously, if you're a slave, you can't say no. But many people, even in relatively free societies, feel powerless to refuse any demand, request or offer. Life, in the form of social conditioning, family dynamics or trauma, has taught them to be helpless, but they think they're being "nice."

People with diabetes and other health problems can't afford to be nice. Imagine Inga has diabetes and goes to a family gathering where her cousin Joan offers her a big piece of homemade cheesecake, "just the kind you love." Joan says or implies her feelings will be hurt if Inga doesn't eat it. People do this kind of thing all the time but Inga can't afford to be nice in this situation.

Or say Marcus is offered a double shift at work. The boss implies that he'd be very grateful, and Marcus knows his family can use the money. But he also knows he needs to rest, he needs to exercise and he needs to eat dinner at the proper time. And he knows he will be best off not telling his boss about his diabetes. Hopefully, Marcus has learned polite, non-revealing but firm ways of saying no.

In situations like these and many others, you can't afford to be nice. I carry a bag of buttons that say, "No more nice girl!" and "No more nice guy!" which I pass out at readings. Buy a book, and I'll throw in a button. Often times, people just want the buttons, because this message is so important to them.

A good self-management or health promotion program will include assertiveness training. Too many people feel they have to do everything for everybody all the time. Such people may be nice to have around, but they're usually not as helpful as they think. They're tired, they're impaired and they're resentful, even if they aren't aware of it. They and those they're trying to please might be better off when they learn to say no and speak up about their real needs and desires. In situations where the power relationships make it difficult to speak up — for example, at work or in the doctor's office — it may help to have other people with them for support.

People have to fight for their health. This doesn't mean fighting diseases like diabetes — illness is just the body's way of trying to cope with toxic conditions. It may mean fighting some of the conditions that cause diabetes. It doesn't usually mean combat either. Some of our strongest weapons are acceptance of ourselves and of others, forgiveness of those who deserve to be forgiven and love for ourselves and the people around us. The best way to battle for your health is to accept and forgive with a fighting spirit.

Reasons to Live

Professionals and media usually tell people that self-care is all about exercise and food. In reality, our health flows from our lives, and anything people do to make their life better, easier or more meaningful contributes to better health. That's why preventing and managing chronic illness often have to start with making people's lives better, not just focusing on health. If parts of people's lives get in their way, we have to deal with those parts.

William Polonsky, Ph.D., author of *Diabetes Burnout* believes that a person's decisions about self-care are based on a cost/benefit analysis.[11] If the benefits of healthy behaviors don't seem worth the discomforts, trouble and expense, people won't practice healthy living. The most commonly cited benefits of diabetes self-care are longer life and avoidance of complications. But the value of those benefits depends on how highly people value their own lives.

If you don't have a reason to get out of bed in the morning, it won't matter how healthy you are. If one's life is filled with stress and pain and has little pleasure or love, why should that person check his blood sugars or avoid donuts, or stop shooting heroin for that matter? Finding reasons to live and reducing the things in our lives that make us miserable, which I call reasons to die, can make a huge difference in our good health.

In a famous study,[12] Drs. Ellen Langer and Judith Rodin divided residents in a Connecticut nursing home into two groups. Each person in each group was given a cheap house plant. One group was told, "We're giving you this plant to make your room look better. The staff will take care of it. Enjoy." The other group got to choose which plant they wanted, and was told something like, "This is your plant. You can take care of it or not, as you choose. It's up to you whether the plant lives or dies." This group was also encouraged to make some other choices, for example, about the arrangement of furniture in their rooms. Eighteen months later, Langer and Rodin were shocked to find that residents in the "just look at the plant" group had died at twice the rate of the group who were taking care of their own plant.

Now, taking care of a cheap house plant is about as minimal a reason for living as you can imagine. But in a nursing home, and in many people's lives, reasons might not be that easy to come by. Imagine a homeless person, sleeping on a cold street, with few friends, no love and no hope that things could ever get better. Why would this person care about controlling their diabetes? So they could live longer? Why would they want to? In some communities, large sections of the population live in situations where the costs of self-care far outweigh the benefits, so the first self-care step is getting some more reasons to live or shedding reasons to die.

It's important to make self-care a positive experience, a reason to live, instead of another burden. Exercise should be fun; it should be convenient and social. A game, a dance, a brisk walk through an interesting environment (like a shopping mall, for some people) can make exercise a source of enjoyment. When it comes to food, it's important to find healthy foods you actually enjoy eating, instead of focusing on the white bread you're giving up.

A major reason to live is quite simply other people. Studies show that isolation is perhaps the biggest reason to die,[13] and loneliness is the biggest risk factor for death among seniors. People's health and health behaviors usually improve dramatically when they become more involved with family or community.

While unemployment devastates many people's health, mainly because of the stress of not contributing anything or having little to do to occupy time, some unemployed people do manage to stay healthy. These tend to be people who get involved in their communities by volunteering and helping others, or who keep life interesting, perhaps by going back to school or getting politically active.

Engaging in self-care and helping others do so, thereby helping protect one's community, is a form of engagement and a reason to live in its own right. In this broad sense, self-care can spread in an ever-widening circle, embracing and healing more and more people. Self-care can become a social norm if people come together to make it happen.

Chapter

7

Strength in Numbers

WHERE DOES THE POWER to fight for one's health come from? The last chapter looked at some internal resources: self-confidence, fighting spirit, and reasons to live. Most people need more, though. They need social support. The best source of power is other people.

Many societies discourage people from seeking, finding or accepting help. We need to resist those social pressures and work together if they are to have a chance of regaining good health. This chapter looks at some of the social barriers to support and the causes of isolation. It describes some ways people can unite for health, and how some new approaches to medical care are bringing people together.

Where Not To Get Help

Needing help has a bad reputation. In America, independence is valued above all else. You're expected to be a John Wayne-type character — strong, silent and completely self-sufficient. Asking for help implies weakness or incompetence. We are raised to think we'll be imposing on people by asking, that we'll be in their debt with no way to repay them.

This personal independence is a myth, of course. Modern society is more interdependent than it ever has been. It is likely that hundreds of people were involved in getting you the food you ate yesterday. When I work with clients and community groups, I tell them that asking for help doesn't mean they're weak; it means they're smart. Most people like to help and don't resent being asked. Helping others makes people feel good about themselves.

The myth of independence has powerful social effects. If we aren't willing to share, then each person requires more, pushing us to consume more. It also places all the responsibility of dealing with hard lives or health problems on the people who have them. A thousand people in a neighborhood could have T2D, and another thousand have alcoholism, and everybody is poor, yet each individual is dealing with it alone. If you were just strong enough or smart enough, if you had enough courage or cared enough, you could rise above the environment and manage your problems by yourself.

As we saw in Chapter 4, standard medical practice reinforces the cultural mandate to go it alone. In the clinic, it's patient and doctor against the world, and in some cases, patient against doctor. Where is the help going to come from?

Help vs. Economics

Families and communities are weakened by economic and social pressures beyond the myth of independence. People move far from their families, often far from their friends and communities. This isolation makes it hard to get help when needed. Economic stress and focus on consumption also drive people away from each other. People may be working too hard to take care of themselves, and they may also stop taking care of each other.

An increase in material consumption can sometimes damage health as well, if it reduces social cohesion. Sociologists studied

Roseto, a community in Eastern Pennsylvania.[1] Made up of close-knit and interlocked Italian families, Roseto had a death rate 40% lower than economically similar communities around them. That advantage lasted from the 1930s to the late 1970s, when people started paying more attention to material standard of living than to family connections. "When Cadillacs started to appear on the roads of Roseto," one researcher wrote, "the health advantage started to disappear." Today, there are few communities like Roseto in the US or in other so-called "advanced" countries. In a society with epidemic levels of isolation, where can people go for support?

The Shelter of Each Other[2]

For most people, family is the most important source of support. A woman named Shelley was diagnosed with T2D at Providence Medical Center in Seattle ten years ago, when she was only 26 years old. With two young children and an abusive husband, self-care had no place on her to-do list. She medicated her stress with food, and her A1C numbers were always extremely high.

Things turned around in two stages. First, her family offered to take her and the children in, and convinced her to accept the offer. Then her beloved father developed T2D too. He became a gung-ho self-care advocate who "drove his family crazy asking us to walk with him," in the words of Shelley's mother. Shelley started to exercise and prepare healthier foods because she "wanted to help her father." Now her blood sugar numbers are down and she feels better than she has in years.

Dr. Catherine Chesla at the University of California at San Francisco has found that "family sense of coherence" is one of the strongest predictors of how someone will cope with diabetes.[3] Families can be the biggest source of stress or the biggest buffer against it. They can facilitate behavior change or block it. Families who support each other and have a sense of working together provide a much better environment for health than households where everyone goes to bed angry.

The first thing health care workers should do for a patient with diabetes or pre-diabetes is ask how the patient's family fits into his life. They should try to bring at least some of the family in for appointments and classes, giving them a chance to get on the same page as the patient. As we know, families of people with T2D are more at risk for getting it too, because they tend to share genes, environments, stresses and behaviors. Patients don't have to wait to be asked, either. They can and should bring their family with them. Don't necessarily stop with the nuclear family; often the extended family can help, so bring them in!

If more medical systems were more inclusive of families, patients would fare much better. But most providers do a poor job of this, or don't even try. There are barriers, of course: some family members don't want to or can't participate. There may be long-term hostilities, stresses or dysfunctions that need addressing. But care providers can save a lot of money and frustration by dealing with such issues — providing or referring families for professional services or other sources of support.

Because family stress, trauma and health problems like diabetes get passed down from generation to generation, supporting families with young children can prevent a lot of future health and behavior problems.[4] But in a society where most insurers are reluctant to pay even for individual prevention, and business plans usually look ahead only one quarter, there is virtually no help for intergenerational prevention.

Building Support into Medicine

The medical system doesn't have to be part of the isolation problem; it can be part of the solution. Some health care systems have found innovative ways to integrate the power of other people in diabetes and chronic illness care. One extraordinarily effective approach is "group appointments" (also called Shared Medical Appointments [SMAs], Cooperative Health Care Clinics [CHCCs] or Drop-In Group Medical Appointments [DIG-MAs]). Instead of seeing patients one by one, a doctor or nurse practitioner has a group of people come in together. Some models prefer groups of 10–16, while other clinics use "mini-groups" of three or four. Families are often invited too.

Practices vary, but I will outline one type of group appointment here. A medical assistant may take vital signs, while a nurse checks patients' feet for signs of skin breakdown or infection. Someone else may review all patients' records to make sure they are up to date on lab tests, vaccinations and other preventative measures. Meanwhile, patients participate in a group discussion, perhaps with a nutritionist about cooking or a diabetes educator about exercise, or, in more forward-thinking clinics, about topics the patients choose. Patients can also have some one-on-one time with the physician if they so desire. The whole process can take anywhere from 90 minutes to three hours. This method (the Cooperative Health Care Clinic or CHCC) usually includes the same group of patients month after month, and works best in a large medical system, where non-physician staff is easily available.[5]

Other versions (DIGMAs and SMAs) are more like one-on-one appointments carried out in sequence while the other patients observe. Psychologist Edward Noffsinger developed these approaches after experiencing the frustration of fighting for access to a traditionally run clinic when he was sick with lung and heart problems. "The one-on-one office visit was way too rushed," he says. "There wasn't time to get my issues and questions addressed, and there were tremendous waits on the phone, in the waiting room, in the exam room, all to get six minutes with the doctor."

Having patients seen in groups has the following advantages, according to Noffsinger: "DIGMAs give people prompt access to care, more time with their own doctor, greater attention to patient education and psychosocial issues. They get answers to questions they never thought to ask, because other patients ask for them. It integrates into each patient's care the help, support, encouragement and suggestion of other patients and also provides closer follow-up care because you can be seen any week you want to."

In Noffsinger's model, a "behaviorist," usually a psychologist or social worker, runs the appointments and manages the sessions. Nurses can also fill this role, and doctors, once they've been trained, can even do it themselves. According to psychologist Vivian Barron of Hill Physicians Medical Group, which includes 2,600 doctors across Northern California, having other patients and families present at the appointments provides benefits no matter what method is used.

"It's the magic of being in a group," Barron says, "and having that amount of time with an M.D. And even if the doctor is very controlling, a patient will say something the doc can't answer, and a patient jumps in and says, 'Well I tried this,' or 'What do you think about that?' They fill in where the physician isn't comfortable."

Research on Groups

The first published report on the group approach came from Turin in northern Italy.[6] In this study, one group of people with T2D received group appointments, while the other received the usual one-on-one care. In spite of having lower educational and economic levels, the group appointment group had far better blood sugars, cholesterol and self-rated quality of life than the traditional care group. The Italians recently published a five-year follow-up showing even greater advantages for the group method in their clinical results. The group patients even reported improved quality of life as their diabetes went on.

Since then, dozens of studies have been published on the group approach. Dr. Dawn Clancy[7], at the Medical University of South Carolina (MUSC), has written about groups she and others lead for uninsured and underinsured patients with diabetes. MUSC has found that patients receive much better care in the group appointment setting (as measured by American Diabetes Association standards), have better results, feel more positive about their clinic visits and have more trust in their physicians.

Patients often fare just as well in non-physician-led group visits. In one study of "cluster visits,"[8] patients met with educators, including a nurse, a dietitian and a pharmacist. Doctors consulted but rarely saw patients. Compared to a primary care control group, cluster visit participants had significantly lower blood sugars, had lower hospital admission rates and reported more self-efficacy related to managing their disease.

What makes group appointments so effective? Rajan Bhandari, M.D., chief of neurology at the Kaiser Permanente Santa Theresa Medical Center in San Jose, says, "[Patients] seem to really blossom when they're in a warm, empathic environment where they feel nurtured, supported and not alone."[9] (Perhaps most physicians don't realize how non-nurturing and unsupportive the usual medical environment is.) Patients are encouraged when they see others coping with problems similar to theirs. It gives them hope, positive role models, contacts and friends who can help one another. Dr. John Scott, who developed the CHCC model, says, "A lot of dynamics happen in a group setting that cannot happen one on one."[10]

Experts were afraid that people wouldn't say what was really on their mind in front of a group, but the exact opposite is often the case. Dawn Clancy says, "In my group, nearly all of them are willing to speak up and ask questions or give advice. A gentleman came in and he wanted to make sure there would be an opportunity to talk privately about his sexual concerns. He didn't want to discuss them in the group. About three months into the group, we were talking about what should be our next month's topic, and he said, 'I think we should discuss sexuality. I think that's very important.'"

Dr. Bhandari says he often discovers things about his patients that he'd never heard before, even though he'd known them for years. "They'll say, 'I feel safe with these five folks here,' or someone else in the group will start talking about something personal, and then they chime in."

Resisting Support

Do groups work for everyone? Some studies show that about one third of patients decline invitations to group visits or do not show up for them, either because they're not comfortable in groups or because the visits last too long. Proponents of the group approach, however, believe that the patient usually hasn't been asked properly. "[Clinics] have problems getting people," says Noffsinger, "because the doctor didn't do the inviting. Would a phone call out of the blue from someone you don't know, pushing something you don't understand, get you to go, or would a personal invitation from the doctor do the trick?"

Some people have psychological issues that may prevent them from joining a group. "Groups don't work for everyone," says Dawn Clancy. "People who did not benefit were people with uncontrolled psychiatric issues or active substance abuse."

However, many people who at first seem too fragile for groups actually benefit from them. "DIGMAs work great," says Jim Deming, M.D. of Mayo Health System's clinic in Tomah, Wisconsin, who even invites patients with schizophrenia to attend. "Patients love listening to other patients' stories. Some patients with significant emotional problems become much more socially appropriate in the group. I am more and more convinced group visits offer something regular visits can't."[11]

Groups and the Medical Model

Group appointments are growing, but they haven't taken over. An American Academy of Family Physicians (AAFP) survey in 2003 found that about 6% of American doctors are currently providing group visits.[12] The roots of resistance to groups must be deep because the group appointments are extremely cost-effective. Despite this, some insurers resist paying for them. In a *Wall Street Journal* article,[13] a spokesman for the insurance company CIGNA is quoted as saying, "We philosophically believe that the patient-physician relationship is a one-on-one relationship, not a twelve-on-one relationship." Notice who is "philosophically" standing up for traditional power relationships.

Yet many other insurance providers pay for groups without much trouble. So where is the resistance coming from? According to Noffsinger, "[The group approach] introduces change at a time where health care systems feel they've changed already. Also, all the hard work gets done up front, preparing the system for the change. Everything gets easier over time, but it's a major paradigm shift."

For some doctors, the hardest part of the new paradigm is having to give up some power. They're no longer the feudal lords ministering to the peasants one by one; they're just the first among equals. But this in itself is a major benefit for all concerned. The groups save doctors' time and energy. Speaking to fifteen people at once is much more efficient than repeating the same thing to fifteen people separately. Physicians often find the groups help them take care of themselves, too. Dawn Clancy remembers one session when she wanted the group to focus on self-testing of blood sugars, but they insisted "We want to lose weight." They started a group exercise program and got the doctor to come along with them, "which I really needed at the time," she says. "I hate to exercise, but they got me going."

Like several doctors I interviewed, Clancy finds the groups save her from burnout and become the high point of her week.

"I left there last Thursday rejuvenated, finally happy again to be practicing medicine. After weeks dealing with residents and all the one-on-one visits, it is just really nice to get together with my group."

Dr. Donald Berwick, leader of the Institute for Healthcare Improvement says, "One-on-one, face-to-face appointments are the dinosaur of the health system."[14] But it's a dinosaur that is hard to kill, as many professionals aren't comfortable working with groups or don't like the idea of giving up their total control over the medical encounter. Bringing patients together in groups increases their power. Often, those who meet in a group become friends and mutual supporters outside of the group. Moving to a group model is one thing the health system can do to help build the movement we need. Patients can help by putting pressure on their health providers to start doing group visits. That should get the ball rolling.

Groups Without Professionals

People with diabetes can come together without a doctor's presence. Diabetes education can and should be given in classes and groups whenever possible, rather than to individuals. Families should almost always be included too. Just as in medical appointments, patients can teach each other, instead of all the knowledge coming from one person.

Good self-management programs, like the ones developed by Kate Lorig and associates at Stanford, are classes with support built into every step. Every session includes two- or three-person activities, group brainstorms and opportunities for group members to give each other feedback. Unstructured break time gives people additional chances to connect with one another.[15]

The use of lay leaders in the Self-Management Program is another source of support. The leaders model the various behaviors the program teaches. Because students know that the teachers face problems similar to their own, they tend to believe that if the teachers can do it, they can too. In self-efficacy terms, this is called "vicarious success."

The Self-Management Program also connects people via a buddy system. People team up and call each other during the week, in between classes, to check up on the other's progress. This process can lead to friendship and ongoing support.

In one Program that I was leading, a woman named Diane told us how her husband had left her with a rebellious teen and two aging parents. She said she didn't have the time for exercise, relaxation or even meal planning. She didn't have enough help. Through the program, however, she met two people who lived in her neighborhood and they started sharing a few meals. One of them worked in her teen's school and started paying attention to him there. Diane began to feel more supported and actually started walking in the neighborhood with one of her new friends.

Support Groups of One

A buddy system is similar to the mentor or sponsor system used by Alcoholics Anonymous and other recovery programs. While few medical providers use this proven resource, some do attempt to hook patients up with one another, and it almost always proves beneficial. In Omaha's Diabetes Education Center of the Midlands, I met two men, Eliot and Morey. Eliot is a self-care fanatic whose business cards list his middle name as NBG, which, he explained, stands for Normal Blood Glucose. When Eliot and Morey met, Morey was struggling to cope with his diabetes. One of the diabetes educators introduced them, and Eliot quickly took Morey under his wing, diabetically speaking. They became close friends. (One Sunday, they took me to the gym where they work out.) Morey's blood sugars are now well controlled, and they're both happy with the relationship.

Most health care providers have long lists of patients they could connect with each other, if they only realized the importance of doing so. Patients who are managing well love to be asked to share their wisdom; it acknowledges their success and expertise. Most health systems just don't consider it part of their job to bring people together, and this needs to change. Again, patients can help by asking for this connection.

Asking for and receiving help is often more powerful than any drug in the treatment of T2D, and people don't have to depend on the health care system for all their help. People with diabetes are everywhere, making support groups a feasible option. They are held in churches, libraries, health centers and senior centers. They not only help a great many people cope with their diabetes, they are also valuable sources of information.

Who Needs Professional Help?

Most diabetes professionals are still caught in the web of power relationships that contribute to diabetes rather than heal it. But individuals, families and communities can find ways to use people power to protect their health.

Social support is why a gym like Curves is so successful. Even though the workout is lighter than most women will find ideal, the act of exercising in a non-judgmental, supportive group keeps women coming back. (I wonder if men can get something like that.) Support is also the key to the success of Weight Watchers. They have succeeded in cultivating the sense that the participants are in it together, that no one is alone and that it is possible to succeed. This feeling helps people maintain health in difficult circumstances.

Churches serve their communities in many ways, and support for diabetes can be one of them, but organized programs, while extremely beneficial, aren't always necessary. Neighbors can also act as support. Finding one exercise partner or getting together with one other person to eat healthy meals might be all someone needs to succeed at self-care.

Escaping the Medical Center

Coming in to a clinic or hospital puts patients at a further power disadvantage relative to their providers. They're on the professionals' turf, surrounded by more powerful people, who are not necessarily on their side. Many people have scary associations and bad memories of previous encounters. They will be more stressed, so less able to learn and change.

If health systems really want to help, their next step after learning to work in groups is to take their services into the community. By getting out of their offices and going where people live, they can lend strength, status, and expertise to a community program. They won't be in complete control, but just like with group appointments, they will enjoy it more and feel a lot more successful.

To help large numbers of people change, to make a difference in the diabetes epidemic, requires change at the community level. We need to change environments as well as behaviors, and more health systems and community activists are recognizing this. In the next chapter, we'll see how people are acting on this understanding, and how it's working.

Chapter 8

Taking It to the Streets

ZIP CODE 97201 is the side of Southern California you never see on TV. In Santa Ana, where citrus orchards once grew, a densely packed city of mostly low-income Latino workers live in big apartment complexes that crowd along the narrow streets. But drivers still speed like they were cruising on country roads.

Not coincidentally, they also have sky-high rates of T2D and overweight children. There's simply no place for kids to be active. "We have one small park," says Caleb Arias, Project Director at Latino Health Access (LHA), a groundbreaking community health organization. "There's a sign there that says 'no active sports.' The schools don't have open space around them, and they don't have money for PE classes. Some of the apartments have outdoor public spaces, but they're posted with signs saying 'No bike riding' 'No ball playing' and 'No loitering.' Kids aren't even allowed to be there."

Out of concerns for kids' safety, parents tell their children to come straight home from school, buy something to eat (usually junk food) from the convenience truck parked outside, go straight into their apartments and stay there until the parents come home. That's an environment highly likely to cause T2D and other chronic problems. So do you treat them with drugs? Do you hope that individuals can somehow change their behavior? Or is there another approach? LHA thinks they have a better solution.

Founded by America Bracho, an M.D. from Venezuela, LHA doesn't treat individuals, it treats the whole community. LHA employs dozens of *promotores* to promote health and fight for a better environment. "We don't choose *promotores*," says Arias, himself a farm worker's son. "They are chosen by community residents. They're the ones who stand up and talk, who communicate from the heart, really speak their minds. They get people motivated enough to say 'We can do this.'"

Dr. Bracho realized that, if people were to get physical, the environment would have to change. And to change the environment, the community would have to be mobilized in other ways. Paid staff and volunteers identified four vacant lots in the district, filthy and garbage-strewn, owned by the city and a local supermarket. Spreading the word at schools and community meetings, LHA developed a core of parents whose support generated the help of a local hospital and some contractors who volunteered their time.

"And we're going to have a park!" says Arias. "But we're making sure that it's a sustainable situation where the parents become the driving force in maintaining the park. It's their park, but they have to take care of it. There will be parents there at all times. It's not going to solve our obesity problem by itself, but that's how things get started, in small increments."

This is a very different way to think about what health care should be and how it should work. It takes health out of the clinic and brings it into the street and into people's homes. It promotes physical activity and healthy eating certainly, but goes beyond individual behavior. It focuses on strengthening community ties and building the power of local people. In this model, health professionals and agencies serve to support the life of a community, not dictate to it.

"We are an institute of community participation and organization," says Bracho. "We aim to organize the talents, resources, knowledge and skills of the community to address the issues they want to address."

Diabetes Care in the Garage

This approach seems far more effective than usual medical efforts. The LHA diabetes self-management program has lowered A1C levels by an average of three points in those who have completed the program, an amazing result. Where might such radical improvements come from?

When Caleb Arias went to his first LHA diabetes class, he was in for a shock. Instead of a clinic or school, the class met in a neighbor's garage. "The garage was really dilapidated," he remembers. "It was used by the tenants to store junk. They set up some folding chairs and some rough wooden benches. People were sitting wherever they could."

The second shock came when he learned who was leading the class. "I see a *promotora*," says Arias, "a person who has diabetes, who has it under control, who lives in that community, who looks like the people in the community, speaks like the people living in that community, teaching the class."

"I knew Sabena had T2D, and it dawned on me, she's leading the class by example. She's letting people know, 'I have diabetes, I went through a process of self-reflection, a journey, and I finally came out at the end of the tunnel knowing about T2D, knowing more about myself, committing to the fact that I had to change the way I live, the way I eat, the way I exercise, because I want to do it for myself. And here I am, and I'm no longer taking medications.' The incredible thing is that all the *promotoras* in this program have T2D, and they're all off meds. It's diet and exercise, and they've been able to stop taking meds."

Other studies confirm that classes led by community members lead to terrific results for the students. In one study sponsored by Pfizer Health Solutions (PHS) — yes, the drug company Pfizer — 1,700 patients enrolled in a program called *Amigos en Salud* (Friends in Health).[1] This was an eight-session course run by local *promotores* or community health workers (CHWs) trained by PHS to "provide patient-centered, culturally appropriate diabetes and depression management." *Amigos en Salud* students have significantly decreased glucose and cholesterol levels, improved diet and exercise and reduced depression compared to traditional care control groups, who took the same drugs, performed the same tests and received the same medical attention.

Interestingly, while the *Amigos en Salud* groups exercised only slightly more and ate just a bit better than the controls, their clinical results were far better than their behavior would have suggested. Although the experimenters haven't analyzed this effect, it was likely the self-efficacy building, stress-reducing effect of community support — having a teacher who was like them, getting together with others to share their problems and successes — that accounted for most of the striking clinical benefits. You probably couldn't get those results if community members weren't leading.

"*Promotores* drive the message home based on the fact that it comes from their heart," says Arias. "This info is available other places. It's the process. It's direct interaction between the *promotores* and the clients, and the clients among themselves."

Community as Patient and Healer

When we think about who gets T2D and why, we realize that communities are wounded and weakened, just as families and individuals are. People are too stressed with economic demands, distracted by consumerism and burdened with feelings of anger, fear, guilt and failure. Jobs and careers push people to relocate frequently. The culture divides us until we're relegated to isolated corners. For too many, "community" is more a nostalgic romantic notion than a real source of support. We are all on our own.

If community is to play a positive role in people's lives and health, it has to be consciously rebuilt and strengthened. For this reason, LHA has begun hiring youth as *promotores*. The youth program began after a project on domestic violence, when adult *promotores* found that residents wouldn't talk with them. "People seemed very afraid," says Bracho, "afraid of each other and of our workers, afraid to go out. They did not want to talk." But the children of the neighborhood did come around. Over the course of one week, the youth brought much of the neighborhood to meetings and a successful anti-violence project was started. Now LHA uses youth *promotores* in much of their work.

LHA's work consistently focuses on connecting people with one another, and connecting the community with the outside world. They have arranged for medical school students to come to the apartments to perform immunizations. They take overweight children to the nearby University of California at Irvine for physical education classes from kinesiology professors and to learn new sports. They hold meeting in schools to encourage parents to get involved.

Why Diabetes?

With all the other problems a community like Santa Ana faces, why should they focus on diabetes? Why focus on health at all, instead of jobs, crime, or other crises? Sometimes other priorities are stronger, but many times a focus on diabetes can empower people for further changes.

Diabetes Educator Martha Funnell, of the University of Michigan's diabetes program, says, "In our work in the inner city, people are so defeated by their lives. For someone who has lost a child to a drive-by shooting, how important can diabetes be at that point in their life? But it's one thing they can gain some control over. They can't control all these financial issues, family issues, the fact that they're raising grandchildren and great grandchildren because parents are not available or able to do that. They want to gain control over something, and starting with diabetes is a place to begin."

America Bracho identifies another reason why her community activists started with diabetes. "The results are easily and directly measurable. If A1C levels come down significantly, you know you're on the right track."

Knowing you're on the right track is healing for everyone. Like individuals, oppressed communities often come to believe they have no power to change things. They have low self-efficacy. "Thanks to the culture's representation of Latinos," Bracho says, "we are immersed in the deficits of our own culture. But when we have success in changing one thing, like with the park or with A1C levels, people get a new sense of their possibilities."

Though they don't use the term, LHA sees community self-efficacy as a goal in and of itself. They arrange for neighbors to meet with politicians and business leaders so residents don't feel ignored by the government. They help *promotores* and others begin to speak out in public and articulate their needs and views to people in power.

Promotores as Organizers

Promotores/CHWs are natural pools of leadership talent. Good community health programs emphasize the creation of new and effective leaders. They choose people who are already outspoken in their church or PTA or neighborhood and train them in communication and meeting facilitation skills before they even mention diabetes. *Promotores* become community organizers.

Vicki Legion, who trains Community Health Workers at San Francisco State University, says, "CHWs have a devoted base and close, warm relationships. So if there's some political thing going on, they are able to mobilize families. The [San Francisco] health department had a $30 million deficit a couple of years ago, and they were going to close the children's asthma clinic. The CHWs got a bunch of families to go out and testify at several hearings, and the health department flipped their position and didn't attack the clinic. People are seeing, 'this is where the decision gets made, and they will listen to me.' It helps people to have those experiences and gain that knowledge."

Partnering

Because few low-income communities have the resources to maintain strong health programs by themselves, organizing involves partnering with governments, congregations, non-profit agencies, health providers, schools, businesses, farmers, anyone. LHA enjoys a lot of media support and political backing in Santa Ana. Their annual Salsa fundraiser is a social highlight.

"It's not just the residents," says America Bracho. "We engage with the businessmen, the builders, the politicians. We need to involve everyone who cares about the future of the neighborhood. If the builders don't come to this neighborhood, if the schools are dismal, if the politicians are not engaged and the businesses do not employ locals, there is no way this community will be a healthy one."

It's also important to partner with doctors and other health professionals. They can provide testimony at hearings and speak at community events. Their proximity to power can make a community feel they have important allies. For many people, their doctor is the most powerful person they know, and it feels good to have him or her fighting on their side.

Athena Philis-Tsimikis is medical director of a program called Project Dulce in San Diego. She says her physicians work well in partnership with communities and other members of a health care team. "Doctors need to be there, but they don't need to be the leaders," she says. "We use nurses, dietitians, diabetes educators and *promotores* who can reach into the community, who understand what people are going through. We use all the pieces together, not one over the other."

Community-based medical care is widely practiced, but the use of clinics as organizing centers is relatively new and still uncommon. It will grow, however, and with it, the wellness movement will too. Non-professionals, however, are already doing some great things, as you'll see in the following sections.

Communities in Motion

Communities, like individuals, often find movement the best way to start health efforts. In the Northwest, the Comprehensive Health Education Foundation (CHEF) rallies groups of seniors together and turns them loose to create self-directed health projects in their communities. One group in Seattle developed a walking program at the local middle school track. They recruited students, many of whom had few adults in their lives, to walk with them. Elders benefited from companionship; students from mentoring; everybody from exercise.

In Oakland, California, a group called 100 Black Men of the Bay Area sponsors programs called Move for Health. "We're trying to revitalize the weekend programs and after-school programs for youth," says Mark Alexander, a Move for Health leader. "These programs have dwindled. A lot of the playgrounds are locked up; the kids don't have safe places to play. There are no funds for structured sports programs. We got together a coalition of volunteers and started youth sports teams.

We actively recruit parents as coaches. We took a small group of kids to the national championships for AAU Junior Olympics this year, based on the track clubs we started in the schools." Move for Health also sponsors intergenerational fitness events like an annual all-day fitness expo in a local park, featuring activities such as youth rock climbing and senior aerobic dance.

Even in the heat of the desert along the Arizona-Mexico border, poor farm-worker communities are eager to get moving, given the right support. Amanda Aguirre, director of the Regional Center for Border Health in Yuma, Arizona, describes their successful walking program. "A *promotora* finds families or individuals who would like to be part of a Walking Club. They provide education on good lifestyles and physical activity, and they structure a series of classes and incorporate neighborhood walking clubs, which are groups of ladies who sign up to walk together. It's very social. They have a graduation festivity and they weigh themselves and they see how well they feel mentally and physically. They see the results. It's very motivating." In the summer, when afternoon temperatures can reach 120 degrees, they walk early in the morning.

Exercise can also improve public safety and community cohesion. In one San Francisco neighborhood, where fear of crime was keeping people indoors, residents got together for regular "safety walks," which made streets safer for everyone. They made contact with troubled local youth, letting them know the adults were watching and were available for help if the young people wanted it. People started coming out after dark and the community became a more pleasant place to live. (Unfortunately this program, which didn't have the support of government grants or agencies, didn't last, which is typical of so many of these programs. They need more social and governmental support, as we'll see next chapter.)

Another way to build safety, community, and activity levels is by accompanying kids on their walk to school. In many places, parents drive children both ways to school, even if it's just a couple of blocks, because they don't feel it's safe for them to walk. The result is out of shape kids, stressed adults and greatly increased traffic and air pollution.

In 1992, in Brisbane, Australia, David Engwicht came up with a solution to all three of these problems—the "walking bus." In a walking bus program, families sign up to walk to school as a group. Usually one parent (the "driver") walks at the front and another parent (the "conductor") at the back. Parents are usually only required to "drive" the bus one or two days per week. Certain corners or houses are designated "bus stops," where students come to be picked up by the walking bus. Sometimes they wear brightly colored slickers or shirts to increase visibility and safety. As students get older and improve their pedestrian skills, they can get off the bus and start walking alone, something that may never happen in places where children don't get walking practice. There's another benefit to the walking bus: people get to know each other and can help each other in other ways, by babysitting for example.[2] In Oxfordshire, England, they have an interesting variation of this idea, for slightly older kids, called the "bicycle train."[3]

Getting Good Food

Access to decent food is a major health barrier for some communities. Karen Rae Ferreira and her husband Antonio started the Indigenous People's Project, which collaborates with the Navajo in Arizona to serve and educate Native Americans who want to live in healthier ways. They began by arranging with a health food company to provide free blue-green algae, a natural supplement, to a group of very low-income people, a program that expanded to 1,500 Native people from over 70 tribes.

Then a Dineh (or Navajo) couple had a vision of sponsoring a Sundance, a sacred ceremonial dance, which would welcome people from all nations and races to gather to dance and pray for

healing. They called this ceremony Little Big Medicine Sundance. "Little Big Medicine means you bring your Little
Medicine, and I bring mine," says Karen Ferreira, "and together
all of us make one Big Medicine. They asked us if we would
come and set up an organic kitchen and a clinic. 2006 will make
our eighth year of service at this Sundance."

Little Big Medicine is big healing, attended by an average of
4,000 people over eight days of dancing and Native spirituality.
"We started small," says Ferreira, "but year after year, we pro-
cure thousands of pounds of organic food. We've provided
14,000–40,000 pounds of organic food in our Sundance
kitchen." They also provide complementary therapies like
acupuncture, homeopathy and massage in their clinic.

People take what they learn at the Sundance and use it to
change their diet and lifestyle year-round. "When we have these
clinics at the Sundance," says Ferreira, "people get familiar with
foods that they really like. Maybe someone really enjoys
quinoa, or some other healthy food. When I ask companies for
a donation of food, I ask them to send literature and brochures
about their product. I give the material to local people who take
it to the grocery store, and say "look, we're trying to eat healthy
food, so I want you to start carrying this and I'll buy it from
you." Every year we go to the local grocery stores, and there are
more and more organic and natural health products in these
stores."

Markets and Co-ops

Small farmers need markets to sell their produce and people in
poor neighborhoods need access to fruits and vegetables.
Farmers' markets are one answer to these needs; they bring the
food to the people. Activists are coming up with new approaches that make farmers' markets more economically viable
and more accessible to more people. In Honolulu, for example,
markets are set up in many different neighborhoods and last

two hours. People come out for their star fruit, bananas and other fruit and veggies. Then the farmers pack up their produce and move on to the next neighborhood.

Food co-ops are another way to make good food available and affordable in rural and poor urban communities. Rural Houston, Minnesota, was left without a grocery supplier when the last private store moved out in the 90s, so the citizens decided to create their own. The Root River Co-op fills a need where there are no other stores. Community members met for years, developed a business plan, raised money from membership fees, lined up low-interest or no-interest loans from community members and opened their store in an empty building provided by the city.

According to experts Greg Lawless and Anne Reynolds, food co-ops need stable leaders who have some knowledge of the grocery business.[4] Without this, food co-ops can easily fail, as they require a lot of work to keep going. Organizers may underestimate expenses or fail to accurately assess members' needs. But co-ops are succeeding all over the world, especially in places where people are already familiar with the cooperative concept.

Thinking Like Organizers

Successful health activists have to think like organizers. Mark Alexander of Oakland's Move for Health learned this the hard way. "At the beginning," he says, "we tried to do this by ourselves. We would sponsor diabetes screenings, for example, and they weren't well attended, no matter how hard we tried to publicize it. So we started collaborating with other groups such as the Black Nurses, the Diabetes and Heart Associations and the churches. We will contact the minister, because if the pastor addresses this issue from the pulpit and encourages the parishioners to get involved, the turnout will be a lot larger. We found that if we were able to engage the gatekeepers of the community, like ministers, principals or union leaders, then we were able to get our message out to more people."

Health care providers can be excellent organizers, because each patient they see may have connections to other community groups. By simply asking patients what their social club is doing about diabetes, or whether their church would like a health speaker, they can move wellness closer to the top of a community's agenda. Clinics and community groups often find creative ways to help each other, if someone takes the lead in bringing them together.

Congregations are one way that communities are already organized. Many of them help members deal with their life issues, including diabetes. The Parish Nursing program in many Catholic parishes enlists volunteer registered nurses, supported by lay Congregational Health Advocates to visit members' homes and hold health events at church.

Some churches have what they call "health ministries," which Christian clergy may note follows in the tradition of Jesus, a healer in the New Testament. "The church is a way to reach people," says one health activist. "They come to the church before they go to the doctor. There are positive role models in the church and they can promote positive lifestyles."

Another aspect of organizing is choosing how many people and how big of an area will best sustain an effective program. LHA started with the 97201 zip code but soon realized that was too big an area. They cut down to block-level organization and finally realized that focusing on one building at a time (with 300–500 residents) was the most effective community approach.

Controlling *Promotores*

One piece of evidence that CHWs/*promotores* are effective is that so many forces are trying to control them. One recurring form of control is requiring certification from a college to be a

CHW. As San Francisco State's Vicki Legion says "Working CHWs feel that if the colleges have a monopoly on testing for competence, they are screwed, because college is not accessible to a lot of poor people. CHWs are nervous about colleges giving out certificates, because in five minutes, they'll say you don't know enough to do the job you've been doing for the last 30 years. We've always said higher education should not have a monopoly on training and certifying; it should just be one avenue."

Limited funding also restricts the use of CHWs. "Community health workers are still very marginalized in the health system," says Legion. "They're usually on grants, and they almost always get laid off. In children's asthma, where everyone would say CHWs are incredibly important, there are probably three permanent asthma CHWs in the US, and hundreds that get laid off when the grant runs out. So one thing is building understanding of their roles and getting them de-marginalized in the health care system." If organizations such as the American Diabetes Association and the American Association of Diabetes Educators became more active in demanding increased funding for CHWs, that would help build the movement. (Both ADA and AADE have published papers supporting the use of CHWs but have not yet done much more.)

How Far Can Communities Go?

Communities can do a great deal to build their strength and reclaim their health. But we can also see the limits. Communities can help people cope and find support, but they find it much harder to address the root causes of illness. Many of the problems affecting people's health are far bigger than what can be changed at the community level. Governments also have to play a positive role to ensure their people are healthy, and there will be widespread battles along the way.

Chapter 9

The Movement Takes Shape

W E'VE SEEN HOW SELF-CARE, medical systems orienting themselves toward self-management, and active communities can make a difference in diabetes. They can help individuals, families and communities to heal. But the forces behind T2D are powerful, and stopping the epidemic will require government to weigh in heavily on the side of wellness. If we want a healthy society, we need a political movement, inside and outside of government, to make that happen.

Where would such a movement start? What are the top priorities, and what is the strategy? For two years now, I've asked everyone I've interviewed, "What would it take for you (or your community, your patients, your people, your country) to get well? What would have to happen?" Although the answers varied in the details, they fall into six categories.

1. Focus on childhood — support parents, children and schools.
2. Social justice — economic, racial and other inequities addressed; people respected and valued.

3. Stronger communities — people help each other and accept help; more connection, less isolation.
4. An exercise-friendly environment.
5. A healthier food environment.
6. A medical system where everyone is covered, with a focus on self-management, wellness and social approaches.

All six points represent different aspects of the same idea. We want a society that values wellness — health, happiness, security, meaningful lives and connection with others — more than it values material gain and consumption. Is that too much to ask? Is it in any way realistic to think about a program that seems so far-reaching, so radical?

The list of needed changes is daunting, yes. Living with diabetes is daunting too, yet millions of diabetics have strong, positive lives in spite of, or sometimes because of the difficulties, because they have committed to personal change. Social change is very similar to personal change: the key is to take one step at a time. The whole program would be best, but any progress helps.

Another similarity between social and personal change: just as having some success at self-care often strengthens individuals to make other changes, a community or a movement that succeeds in one area may likewise go on to other successes. And there are other similarities. Committing to self-care and social change are both valuable in and of themselves, whatever the results. The commitment makes people better and stronger, bringing strength to the people around them. There is nothing to lose by trying.

Starting with Self-Care

The movement for wellness can't be separated from other movements in the modern world. Wellness is incompatible with poverty and oppression, so it's a social justice issue. When

we talk about healthier food, we are also talking about supporting small farmers and organic farmers who grow most of it.
Promoting physical activity means getting people out of cars,
doing more of their own work and having more of their own
fun. The results could be energy savings, cleaner air and water,
fewer wars for oil and fewer people with T2D.

Strengthening communities and focusing on children will
address a wide range of problems, from crime to cancer, by reducing stress and isolation. A socially just and more equal economy will also be a stronger economy, as well as one that makes
people healthier. Because of the wide-ranging benefits, the
Diabetes Wellness movement can gain support from most of
society.

But, I'll say it again, the movement has to start with self-care.
As Dr. Melanie Tervalon, co-founder of the Health Conductors
movement in Alameda County's African-American community
says, you can't tell other people to do something you're not
willing to do yourself. Further, as self-efficacy theory shows,
when people do the best they can for themselves, they will
tend to be more confident and courageous about confronting
those in power about their needs or the needs of their children.
Being in better shape gives people more energy to fight for
change.

Dr. Tervalon and others started the Health Conductors in
the "spirit of Harriet Tubman," a leader on the anti-slavery Underground Railroad in the 1850s. "Harriet took us from slavery
to freedom and never left anyone behind," says Tervalon.
"[Health Conductors] is taking people out of poor health, into
full wellness in mind, body and spirit."

The Health Conductors meet in groups of three, or trios,
and commit to making specific health-related behavior changes.
They support each other in maintaining their changes. From
that basis in self-care, the Conductors take the message to the
larger community. They volunteer at community-related health

activities, speak at family or community meetings on health and commit to joining and being active in a community health initiative. Once a month the Conductors have general meetings, attended by over 200 people. Each trio tells the group what they have been doing. "The teaching that happens there kind of blows you away," says Tervalon, "because there's so much creativity in what people do."

The Health Conductors recognize that the stress of powerlessness and hard lives makes wellness a much more difficult goal. They address this problem with an emphasis on stress reduction through the practices of meditation, yoga, tai chi and group support. For people struggling with the strains of racism, poverty and everyday life, these practices can provide valuable assistance.

Self-care is extremely important, but it is only a starting point. "As a Conductor, your responsibility is not only to take care of yourself, but to recruit other Conductors," says Tervalon. "Then become a health activist in your church, at your job, on your street. We see it as a way to rebuild the links in the African-American community around our sense of community and well-being."

The movement is also clearly about building leaders, giving people speaking experience and encouraging them to go out and promote health in a wider circle. Each trio has a "guide," and each guide has from five to twelve trios, who together make up a conductor "line." Supported by the Bay Area Black United Fund, the California Endowment, the Alameda Public Health Department and others, the leadership hopes to enlist 4,650 Health Conductors (1% of the Black population) in the seven Bay Area counties. They hope 1% will be the "critical mass" where healthier lifestyles become the community norm. They also expect that the Conductors' self-care plans will grow to include changing their environment and empowering their community.

Supporting Self-Care

Led by activists or health care workers, self-care movements are occurring in hundreds of communities. But we know that the demands and enticements of modern society, especially around food, stress and physical activity, are hostile to self-care. One percent may not prove a critical mass at all, given the powerful forces trying to hold it back.

If health care systems support the self-care efforts, though, these efforts will have a much better chance of sustaining. The self-management paradigm is spreading through medical systems worldwide, led by visionaries like health educators Kate Lorig and a growing army of reformers. Funders and facilitators, such as the Institute for Healthcare Improvement, the Robert Wood Johnson Foundation, the Kellogg Foundation and many statewide organizations such the California Healthcare Foundation and its analogs in many states, are supporting their work. These leaders may well reach the tipping point in Western medicine, where self-care will be acknowledged as primary and providers will seek to build patients' capacity for self-care instead of working to reinforce medical power. The self-management movement is still young, however, and it may be some time before it comes to your local medical center, unless you ask for it, loudly.

Although most are still run in the top-down medical model, some community clinics and visiting nurse associations are bringing self-care support to their neighborhoods.[1] If people hear the same self-care message in their community and from the medical system, that will help, but it won't be enough. Fortunately, there is more. Some businesses have set up wellness programs, with the understanding that healthy employees work better and take fewer sick days. Xerox Corporation reported a five-fold return on investment from their employee fitness program.[2] Such programs are widespread in Japan and are spreading internationally. But for long-term, widespread self-care success, we have to change the way society approaches health, making healthy living easier. For that, we'll need the help of government.

Reclaiming Public Health

Promoting the people's health and wellness has been a role of government for centuries. Public health programs have brought better health to more people than all the doctors who ever lived put together. Government-sponsored efforts have cleaned up the water and air, vaccinated children, helped feed the malnourished, greatly reduced smoking and more. Most of these advances occurred because people fought for them and pushed government to make some changes. There is no reason public health can't address the environmental problems surrounding food, inactivity and stress that contribute to T2D. But for that to happen, public health must return to its roots.

"Public Health Departments (PHDs) were never about the delivery of medical care," says Kimi Watkins-Tartt, acting director of Community Health Services in Alameda County. "We have always been about creating a healthier environment, improving social determinants of health. But we've become the health care provider of last resort. If you can't get medical care, we'll open up a health clinic and we'll provide it. So all of our funding is going to medical care and individual case management and behavior change services, and that will only take you so far. We are now working to get back to our traditional role. We participate in transportation planning meetings. We meet with urban planning and ask questions. 'Why would you build [a city] that way? There are no sidewalks, nobody can walk.' They used to look at us like, 'Why are you here?' But now they understand that what they do is a big part of health."

Governments can collaborate with community groups. This kind of partnering is usually more productive than government doing the work themselves. In Alameda, the PHD set up diabetes working groups made up of community residents and organizations. With PHD support, the working groups have set up farmers' markets in poor neighborhood and walking clubs in local churches. PHD has helped other neighborhoods open parks and make improvements to traffic safety so children can walk without being afraid. The process has also strengthened major skill sets of the participants: community groups gained experience with grant funding, and individuals learned valuable leadership skills. Public health workers call this "building community capacity," the same language self-management experts use in talking about patients' capacity for self-care.

Activity programs can also be implemented at the local or state level. Indianapolis has a publicly sponsored, multi-faceted program called "Indy in Motion."[3] "Colorado On The Move" is a statewide example.[4] England has a national Bike Network devoted to creating safe, appealing places to ride.[5] Creating public places to move and exercise is a common area for government/community partnership and an ideal place for a wellness movement to build strength, because there's no opposition. In theory, at least, nobody is against exercise.

Setting Limits

Governments can and should support positive efforts, but they have another important role: setting limits on harmful activities. Localities or states could act to protect children from unhealthy food in stores and schools and to promote physical activity, and some jurisdictions have done so. They could put healthy food in their food programs and not let food stamps be used for sugary foods. They could mandate that developers make new communities safe for walking and biking; they could require creation of walking and biking trails that go places people actually want to go.

One way to make this happen is through people pressure. In Yuma, Arizona, as in thousands of other places, safety has been a big barrier to exercise. "We have dark streets, with no lighting, no safety walks, no walking paths," organizer Amanda Aguirre says. "Can I go out and walk in the streets and not be mugged? Or not be found by a gang? So we got to the City Council and convinced them to invest in a well lit walking path. Some of the park areas are now better lit, and the loose dogs are more confined."

Lobbying and pressuring politicians has had some powerful results. The food labels on American packaged food didn't come about by industry's public-spiritedness or politicians' concerns about health. They resulted from 20 years of political effort led by activist citizens and health scientists. Activism has also led to the great decrease in cigarette smoking in the last 25 years.

Standing outside the walls of government and shouting has its limits, though. Sometimes you have to get inside, as Amanda Aguirre has done. She is now a state representative with growing influence. On a typical day she may educate local school boards about nutrition and push for a physical education program in schools, advise the Arizona Dairy Council about school nutrition policy and meet with the Latino Caucus on diabetes policy recommendations. At the policy level, she has worked with the State Medicaid Agency and the State Health Department about funding programs and adequately reimbursing doctors in rural areas.

Health workers are often pushed into running for office or accepting appointments because the system they work in seems to be failing. Judy Biros Robson sought election as a Wisconsin State representative when she became frustrated by policies that would pay for seniors' expensive ambulance trips to Emergency Rooms, but not for the home nurse visits that would have prevented the emergency in the first place. She ran as an extreme underdog, but found, as others have, that nurses are widely respected, trusted and electible.[6] Perhaps the presence of more health workers and activists in government could be a big step toward a healthier world.

There are health-conscious legislators and officials already in place. New York State Assemblymen Jimmy Meng and Felix Ortiz of Brooklyn have proposed health-related laws in the legislature and led marches for health in the community.[7] The public needs to offer support to leaders like these, and encourage them to broaden their focus beyond simply behaviors to the social causes of illness.

Saving the Next Generation

For several reasons, the most important step beyond self-care is fighting to protect children. People will often do things for their children they wouldn't necessarily do for themselves. It's harder to put the blame for unhealthy behavior on young children, so there is more openness to government intervention on their behalf. From a medical point of view, prevention is much more effective than treatment. Dr. J. Fraser Mustard, a founder of the Canadian Institute for Advanced Research, says, "We know that a child subject to deprivation or stress is far more likely to experience mental illness, obesity, Type 2 diabetes, heart disease and a shortened life span. So support to families with children is essential." If we support families during a child's infancy or even before it is born and continue this all the way through school, providing good schools and good child care, we will prevent numerous health and social problems.

Although some moralizers want to punish young parents under the slogan of "personal responsibility," you can't actually help children without helping parents. If pregnant mothers are undernourished, or have high levels of blood sugar from a bad diet or their own T2D, the child will be much more likely to be overweight and to contract T2D. If parents are stressed, the child will likely have high levels of stress as well, perhaps for life. If children are not breast-fed, they are also more likely to get T2D.

In 1995, the University of Otago in Christchurch, New Zealand, joined with community representatives to create the Early Start program.[8] Disadvantaged families were eligible to receive free visits from trained support workers for up to five years. Early Start has demonstrated a wide range of health, developmental and behavioral benefits, everything from better school attendance to fewer accidents.

Professor David Olds of the University of Colorado has demonstrated in several studies that having nurses visit pregnant mothers and teach parenting, encourage breastfeeding and provide emotional support led to advantages for the children. The visits continued for the first six months of the baby's life. The children he first worked with are in third grade now and still doing better in several measures of health and behavior than the control group, which did not receive the home visits.[9] The mothers also reported less difficulty coping with life stresses. It is likely that reducing parental stress will hold these kids in good stead for a lifetime. The Nurse Family Partnership that Olds' team created is still active and connecting with community organizations around the country.[10]

Other groups have placed paraprofessionals or lay people in the parental-support role with good success. Helping young families with child care, preschool and sometime financial support also makes a big difference. And how about giving young adults regular support before they get pregnant in order to avoid this situation? Supporting parents and children is a job for communities, but government needs to sponsor it. Community health agencies and visiting nurse associations, church groups and neighborhood organizations like Latino Health Access could carry out such programs, but only if they were funded and mandated.

Schools also make a big difference. They can promote health or promote illness. To be a positive force, they too need more outside support. Good preschools and schools greatly increase lifetime productivity and encourage better health. That's why most industrialized countries in the world (except the US) provide low-cost or free, high-quality preschool for children regardless of family income.[11,12]

Schools can and should teach healthy living. In the CATCH (Coordinated Approach to Child Health) program, schools are supported by state and federal governments to increase students' physical activity and serve healthier food. Since these changes typically cost money and involve behavior change from school staff, CATCH requires dedicated implementers at each school site. This program is strongest in Texas, where Texas Department of State and Health Services pays for the implementation. California, Louisiana, Minnesota and other states also participate in CATCH programs.[13]

Schools can actually become engines of health. Frick Middle School in Oakland suffers all the problems of a school in a poor, mostly African-American and Latino neighborhood. School achievement was low, discipline problems were high and health was awful. Kids were overweight, out of shape, on the way to T2D. Then Principal Calvin Criddle brought in Kermit Bayless, a boxing coach with an education credential, to make physical education "the heart of the school." Students participate in disciplined, high-energy callisthenic and aerobic exercise for 55 minutes at least four days a week. Students now pass the California fitness test at a 68% rate, compared to 29% statewide. Behavior has improved. Academic scores have gone up 45% in five years.[19] The whole community gets involved in Frick sports events. Health, good behavior and achievement tend to go together. We could use more examples like Frick and fewer schools where students are required to sit quietly all day.

Changing the Diet of Death

High-sugar foods are everywhere, and they're spreading. They are promoted heavily to children, with Walt Disney characters appearing on cereal boxes and sports stars promoting soft drinks.[14] Sodas and sweet snack foods are sold in school vending machines and advertised in cafeterias. Meanwhile, fruits and especially vegetables are often hard to come by. In this sugar-saturated society, what chance does healthy eating have?

One important step is making healthy food more available. The Monterey County Farm to School Partnership Program[15] in northern California supports small farms while bringing produce to children. "We connect schools with local farms," says Farm to School director Kari Bernardi. "We provide locally grown farm-fresh fruits and vegetables in the cafeterias, but also the hands-on experience of school gardens, where children can get familiar with different kinds of foods. We find they're more likely to eat them if they have grown them or know what they are."

Growing food has advantages for nutrition, physical activity and community building. Bernardi says she is constantly struck by how gardens help people grow. "We have kids who have been working in their school garden for the last three years," she says, "and over and over we hear them saying, 'We work as a team here.' This is in a neighborhood that's infested with gangs. 'But here in the garden we work as a team.' I just think that's beautiful. That's real social change."

Any school can run a program like this; "gardens" can simply be indoor pots if there is no outdoor space. Bernardi writes grants for stipends to bring farmers into the classrooms, so students appreciate farming as a valued occupation. "We try to bring a healthier diet to the children, but also a healthy, vibrant economy to our local farmers," says Bernardi. This would be a lot easier if governments funded such programs regularly, instead of organizers having to hustle grants from year to year.

Farm and food activists like Bernardi are valuable parts of the diabetes movement. Supporting small farmers is critical to maintaining food quality and diversity, which in turn promotes healthy eating that prevents diabetes. Because food and agriculture corporations increasingly squeeze farmers out or take them over, healthy produce becomes less and less available.[16] Similar programs to the Farm to School Program are being run in colleges — Cal State Monterey Bay coordinates Monterey County's program — and even jails. Growing food for local schools and soup kitchens seems to have a healing effect for some convicts and may lead to jobs upon release.[17] Canada has a national office of urban agriculture to promote healthy food cultivation, as do many cities in the US.

Limiting Poison

Bringing in good food helps, but limiting seductively packaged and promoted poison is also an important step in stopping diabetes. Psychologist Kelly Brownell is director of the Yale University Center for Eating and Weight Disorders. In his book *Food Fight,* he advocates a number of measures to create a healthier food supply. Here are just a few of them:

- Stop marketing food to children.
- Protest and pressure companies and celebrities who lend their names and characters to promoting unhealthy food to kids.
- Level the playing field so healthy foods are promoted at least as much as unhealthy foods.
- Tax food ads, or put small taxes on unhealthy foods to subsidize healthy foods and wellness programs.
- Ban unhealthy food promotions and sales in schools.
- Fund schools adequately so they are not driven to sell and promote bad food to run their programs.

Another important step would be for government to stop subsidizing the production of sugar and grain and the opening of fast-food restaurants and liquor stores. Currently, small business loans and support programs for minority and woman-owned businesses frequently pay for businesses that damage the communities in which they operate. We might also consider banning or sharply limiting the use of high-fructose corn syrup, the chemical sweetener that adds more calories to food at less cost than any other.

As bad as some of the environmental and health effects of modern food industries are, we cannot paint the industry as all bad. We can't knock them for making food cheap, especially when millions of people still can't find enough to eat. From the health perspective, food marketing is what's at fault, not food production. (From an environmental perspective, you could attack both.)

In fact, food insecurity — not knowing whether you'll have enough to eat — is a major risk factor for overweight and T2D. Both behavior and metabolism change when food supply is problematic.[18] People who have experienced famine (or had parents who experienced it) will tend to eat more when they can, simply because it is there, and their bodies will become more insulin resistant and store more fat in preparation for the possible next famine. A wellness movement would focus on food distribution as well as food quality, another place where social justice, the environment, and health come together.

Building for Active People

Modern societies, especially in the US, Canada and Australia, are built for cars, not people. As more people worldwide spend more time in cars, the rate of T2D and other chronic illness is exploding. If developers and automakers paid the health costs associated with their products, they would have to charge a lot more for their goods. If potential home buyers considered the health effects of their residence choices, the landscape would look much different. People would live within walking distance of places to work and shop; pedestrians would be safe crossing the streets. People might stay in town instead of moving ever outward in an automobile-dependent sprawl that damages the environment and people's health. Government should mandate exercise-friendly development, tax excessive sprawl, make streets, parks and public transportation safe and accessible, and perhaps subsidize exercise facilities at work and in school.

Medicine that Heals

We have seen how medical systems can damage health and how they can promote it. To promote it, the most important thing health providers can do is encourage self-management and build self-efficacy. They can help bring people together as we saw in Chapters 7 and 8. They can also play a political role in organizing and advocating for people. Nineteenth century pathologist Rudolph Virchow said, "Physicians are the natural attorneys of the poor." This "attorney" role can often prove more important and helpful than their clinical expertise, which in chronic illness is often of limited value. Because of their respected social position, physicians are more likely to be heard by a school board considering soft-drink vending machines or a legislature considering funding preschools. Physicians can't necessarily be expected to find such opportunities on their own, but they can put their higher status at the service of other parts of the movement, if they receive some leadership and see advocacy as part of their job.

Community health workers are another powerful potential force. As Vicki Legion of San Francisco State says, "Health workers of all kinds can be very active in critiquing the unhealthy conditions of society because they are up against it all the time." Community nursing operations and clinics can help people organize, if they understand community empowerment as an important goal.[1]

Everyone needs access to health care, which in the US means a large expansion of government coverage. To be economical and effective, the health system needs to be based on empowerment, wellness and social approaches. To make such health care available and affordable, society will need to accept limits to what medicine can do in terms of fabulously expensive technological treatments.

Taking the Biggest Step

Committing to self-care, changing the food and activity environment and shifting the focus of medicine to a self-management approach would make a big difference in people's health and wellness. We can count on that; but we also know that bigger problems and challenges, if unaddressed, will limit our capacity to change, and we will be left to simply nibbling around the edges of a much bigger problem.

We have to change the powerlessness too many people have, or feel they have, and we need to rebuild and strengthen communities and families. We live in a society that has gone badly wrong in several ways; the T2D pandemic is only one of them. A wellness-based movement can make a big difference in these other areas, too — the environment, social justice, decreasing violence — and I want to close with a vision of the future that such a movement might bring.

Chapter 10

Diabetes as a Turning Point

"Hope is like a road in the country.
There never was a road,
but when many people walk on it,
the road comes into existence."

— LIN YUTANG

WITH COMPLICATIONS OF DIABETES ravaging his body, an Ojibway man returns from the city of Winnipeg to his tribal land and takes up some of his people's traditional ways. He confronts and comes to terms with the traumas and losses his people have suffered and the losses he has personally endured. He stops some harmful habits and starts to take care of himself. His attitude changes; his feelings change. He becomes whole. He begins to help others.[1]

This is the story line of a Canadian documentary film called "The Gift of Diabetes;" many people with T2D have similar stories. Diabetes can be a wake-up call, moving people toward a healthier, happier, more meaningful way of life. The response to diabetes is the turning point, not the disease itself. If people accept the challenge, find the support they need and take more control of their lives, those with chronic illness can become a source of strength, inspiration and support for a family or a community. They can be a force for positive change.

As I've mentioned before, personal change is not so different from social change. Could a positive and active response to diabetes and chronic health conditions be a turning point for families, for entire communities, even for the world? Could such a response help create societies of people who take care of themselves, of each other and of their environment, instead of pursuing material gain, power and instant gratification? This is what it would take to stop diabetes. Could a movement growing up in response to diabetes move us toward a society which values wellness and community? In which everyone is valued, everyone is responsible, everyone is supported? There are encouraging signs that this transformation could happen.

Stopping or controlling T2D will involve profound social, environmental, economic and political changes. This is an awesome challenge, but one that could bring wonderful benefits. Each of these changes would help millions of people in myriad ways. Each change already has a large constituency. A movement for wellness could be a way of uniting these causes and the people who care about them.

We saw in the last chapter some political approaches people are taking, or could take, to improve food and exercise environments and support parents and children. We saw how people are committing to self-care and to health promotion in their communities. Can we go beyond this kind of local activism to challenge the massive inequalities, power disparities, environmental destruction and materialism that cripple communities and create chronic illness? How could we make that happen? How could a wellness approach help?

Reducing Inequality and Insecurity

Richard Wilkinson, sociologist author of *Unhealthy Societies*, Paul Farmer, physician author of *Where There Is No Doctor*, and others have written extensively on the relationship between inequality and illness. Research shows that greater inequality leads to higher levels of illness. Inequality is built into the structure of national and global economies. Wage levels, tax codes and subsidies are all structured to increase inequality, as wealth produced by some people in some places is sent to far places and given to other people. Day in, day out, the world economy redistributes wealth from the poor to the wealthy.

Governments could reduce inequality and promote health by such changes as raising minimum wages, changing tax policies to be more distributive and guaranteeing or encouraging full employment. Measures to diminish or eliminate racism and other forms of discrimination would also make a profound difference.

Some social scientists dispute Wilkinson's thesis about how inequality affects illness levels. They argue that the degree of inequality is not as important as the degree of insecurity. If the social ladder is steep, it is true that those nearer the bottom will feel a greater stress because of their lack of power. But if food, housing and medical care were guaranteed, the stress would be much less. If good schools were guaranteed from preschool through to college, people would have hope, which prevents depression. It may be that strengthening and raising the safety net is a less controversial approach than trying to make income levels more equal. Either approach would help a great deal.

Especially healing would be self-determination and empowerment for oppressed people, especially indigenous peoples and African-Americans. These folks suffer from disproportionately high rates of almost every chronic illness and social problem. They are treated with a vast array of "services" — medicine, counseling, welfare payments, social work and more — provided mostly by people in the dominant community, often the people who caused the problems in the first place. These services aren't nearly as helpful to oppressed people as gaining power over their own communities and lives would be. Taking on this challenge provides another direction in which the wellness movement could grow and be effective.

Rebuilding Family and Community

Changes will be more effective if implemented in a community-based way. If the government is simply handing out checks, then isolation and lack of support will continue unabated, or even worsen; this is a band-aid solution. The culture of individualism and the striving for material goods are health hazards in and of themselves. We need to rebuild community to get people used to helping and accepting help. The community activists we met in Chapter 8 are promoting such change. Health providers can, too. In rural Alabama, a project was funded to maintain the independence of elderly persons. Because organizers listened to community voices who wanted to include the whole community, the project became intergenerational. Volunteer coalitions developed to address the needs of the elderly, create after-school and summer tutoring programs for children and establish a school-based community health center.[2] Other community groups and the political advocates of community, such as the Green Party and the Communitarians, could support such efforts and help to build the movement.

Obviously, large-scale social and economic changes won't come solely from local efforts like walking clubs or school-based diabetes prevention programs. We need more power than that. Groups will have to come together across divides of place, interest, race/ethnicity and class. We'll have to think nationwide and worldwide. I choose to believe this kind of thing is possible, because researching this book has taught me the power of hope.

The Power of Hope

In writing this book, I have been blessed in meeting scores of inspiring people. I knew going in that living with chronic illness is frustrating and frightening. So is having a lot of it in your family or community. Even working with diabetes can be a source of sorrow and anger. But so are all the other emotional issues, health problems and social problems that people, especially disempowered people face. And so are the issues that threaten all of us — wars, environmental destruction, climate change and more. But the people you have read about here haven't given up the fight, or given up hope.

We live in a time of crisis. Diabetes isn't the crisis; it's just one symptom of it. In very general terms, I'd say the crisis is that a relatively small number of people are consuming huge amounts of resources and doing so through violence and the threat of violence. And the vast majority of people are going along with the destructive status quo, either out of ignorance, or because they're blinded by the consumer culture, or because they have to. But we can't give up. Giving up means betraying our children and ourselves, and giving the world to people who don't love it and don't deserve it. I would like to close with a quote from one of the most inspiring people I've met on this journey, America Bracho.

"In order for people to have hope, they must believe that they can make a difference, that they can influence change in their lives and the lives of others. These changes do not have to be large, they do not have to be spectacular. Hope can grow in the smallest of cracks. It is only necessary for people to take part in a project and to witness the changes it brings. If hope begins to take root, then anything will be possible."

That's the kind of medicine that can make a difference, and we can all practice it. There are dozens of ways to participate, but there are requirements, as the Health Conductors put it. You have to commit to taking care of yourself, to being courageous in advocating for health, to asking for and accepting help, and allowing Spirit into your life. I think we can all handle that. Get involved in the movement; or realize that you're already part of it. Be good to yourself, and I look forward to meeting you some day along the barricades.

Appendix

Self-care

A DIABETES SELF-CARE MANUAL needs more than one chapter. If you're new to diabetes or have never taken it seriously before, you will need more than this Appendix. The Resource List will give you some ideas. (The note numbers [1] correspond to items in Notes, found on page 189.) You can learn more from books,[2] web sites,[3] a diabetes educator,[4] doctor, community health worker or diabetes support group.

In this section, I focus on information and ideas you can't easily get in other places. You'll get tips on developing an exercise program you can actually stay with, how to know what to eat, and complementary treatments you might want to try. You will learn about the barriers to self-care and how to overcome them. Hopefully, you will gain a better sense of control and some new sources of support.

What Diabetes Self-Care Includes

In my books, workshops and lectures, I say self-care includes anything that makes your life better or easier. Any time you pay more attention to the needs of your body, mind, and spirit, you are engaging in self-care. Anything that reduces the demands and stresses of life will help you stay healthier, and counts as self-care. So will anything that gives your life more enjoyment, meaning, and purpose.

Most professionals don't take quite that broad a view. The American Association of Diabetes Educators (AADE) has developed a list of the "Seven Self-Care Behaviors."[5] The AADE 7 are:

- Healthy eating.
- Being active.
- Self-monitoring.
- Appropriate medication use.
- Problem-solving.
- Emotional coping.
- Risk reduction — like quitting smoking.

This list is a great start, but they left out a few important things, including relaxation, positive goals, communication skills and assertiveness. You will learn ideas in all these areas in this Appendix.

Barriers to Self-care

The AADE 7 all involve behavior change — different ways of thinking and acting, and we all know that such changes are easier said than done. There are two basic reasons why behavior change is so hard.

First, our brains are programmed to keep doing what they've done before. We are all creatures of habit. Every time you do an action or think a thought, the nerve cells involved in triggering that behavior get stronger. They gain more of the chemicals they need to transmit messages in the future. They grow new connections (synapses) to send their messages even more forcefully. For this reason, you can't actually break habits. They're hard wired. But you can replace a habit with another, stronger habit. So behavior change is all about forming new habits.

The second, more powerful barrier is that our environments are set up to support our current habits. If you already have a car, it's faster and easier to drive than take the bus, walk, or bike. It's hard to find social support for dealing with stress, but self-medication with food or alcohol is as easy as going to the kitchen. If you smoke, you know where the cigarettes are and whom you can light them around. You might not know what you would do with yourself if you quit. When it comes to taking time for self-care, the environment is generally hostile, as we saw in Chapter 6. These are formidable obstacles to change.

Keys to Self-care Success

What do people need to succeed at behavior change? Four things:

- Self-confidence — the belief that you can do the change.
- Hope — the belief that the change will do some good.
- Motivation — positive reasons to live, belief in your own value.
- Social Support.

It's also important that the changes you want to make fit in with the rest of your life, your values and beliefs.

Two key methods in behavior change are "goal setting" and "action planning." In self-management training,[6] a goal is something you'd like to accomplish over the coming weeks or months. It could be a health goal. ("I want to lower my A1C to 7%.") It could be a fitness goal, like being able to walk two miles or climb the stairs without getting out of breath. Or it could be a life goal, like being able to play with your grandchildren, get a dog, or go back to work. It can be anything that will make your life significantly better.

If no goal jumps out, I often have people in my classes answer a few questions. "Is there something you would like to do that your condition prevents you from doing?" "What would make you excited about getting out of bed in the morning?" "What's the most important thing in your life now?" "What do you want more than anything else now?" "What does your body seem to want from you now?" It's OK, desirable in fact, to get help from loved ones, friends, or professionals in developing your goals.

Your goal should be for the medium term. If you've been sedentary, running a marathon is not medium-term. Maybe in the long-term you can do it, but whatever your goal, you want to break it down into chunks of a few weeks to months.

Your goal doesn't have to be strictly health-related. A lot of times people have needs and priorities that block self-care, and those may need to be addressed first. You can use goal-setting and action planning for any type of life change, but the goal shouldn't be health-destructive.

One Step at a Time

Your goal is a motivator, something you work toward. The steps you take toward your goal are called "action plans." The action plan is a contract you make with yourself — one specific activity that you are going to do in the coming week. An action plan must be:

1. Something you WANT to do — not necessarily something the doctor told you to do, or something you think you SHOULD do. Wanting to do it puts some energy behind it.

2. Something you reasonably CAN do. It's better to say you'll walk three days this week and do it, than to plan for five days and do four. The first way builds self-confidence and sets the stage for further growth. The second way makes you want to give up.

3. A specific behavior, not an outcome — You can control behavior, not always outcomes. "I will limit ice cream to one serving/week," not "I will lose weight." Make it specific. What, where, when, how long, how often, with whom? Sample: "This week I will walk 4 times, for 30 minutes at a time, around the block, after dinner, with my dog."

Say your goal involves getting in better physical shape, and you have decided to take up swimming. You might need to find a pool you like and can afford. You'll need a bathing suit. You might want to arrange swim lessons or find someone to swim with. All of these could be the subjects of action plans. ("This week I will visit two thrift stores that sell bathing suits and buy at least one.") If you've got all the preliminaries covered, you might make a plan to actually swim. ("This week, I will get in the pool 3 times for 30 minutes at a time and swim vigorously at least half that time.")

One key to building self-confidence is to actually succeed at something you want to do, even if it's a very small step. You can maximize your chances of success with a "confidence level" (CL). On a scale of 1–10, how confident are you that you can complete the action plan? It's not the fraction of the action plan you will do. It's how sure you are of completing the entire plan. Your CL has to be at least 7, preferably 8, otherwise you can be pretty sure you won't do it. If your CL is less than 7, ask yourself, what might get in the way of completing this plan? How could I overcome those barriers? What would get my CL up to 7? Sometimes, you have to problem-solve solutions to the barriers (like finding child-care so you can go to the pool. It's OK to get help with these barriers). Other times, you have to make the plan easier (like saying you'll go twice this week instead of four times). When you've got your CL up to 7 or 8, you've got yourself a plan.

The sample form on the next page shows how it looks in practice.

Sample Action Planning Form

Date: _____

This week I will _____
(type of activity)

I will do this _____ times for _____
(time or amount of activity)

I will do this (when, where, with whom?):

_____

_____

_____

On a scale of 1–10, my confidence that I will complete the entire plan is _____

Things that might get in the way of this plan are:

_____

_____

_____

Ways I might overcome these problems are

_____

_____

_____

I carried out my plan on the following days:

MON	TUE	WED	THU	FRI	SAT	SUN

NOTES (anything interesting that happened):

_____

_____

_____

_____

_____

The idea is to move from success to success. Each week, you might build to a higher level or maintain your current level, or add something completely different that might help you toward your goal. You might have to start slowly and build up slowly, but this process can take you anywhere you want to go.

I had a very heavy client whose starting exercise plan was to walk to the mailbox in front of her house each morning. That was all she could do. Then she would rest a while before returning to the house. She slowly built up until she was walking three miles a day! She lost some weight, and her blood sugars are better controlled. It took her a year to get there, but that year was going to go by anyway. So start from wherever you are, and you will probably be surprised at how much better you can get.

Let's Get Moving

So where do you want to start? You can choose from the AADE 7 or anything else that is important to you. This Appendix includes several health-promoting behaviors. You will probably see a lot of things you're doing right already and a few you'd like to change. Pick one or at the most two to start with. Don't make yourself crazy trying to do too many changes all at once, or the changes won't stick.

That said, I'll start by talking about physical activity. Insulin resistance is best cured through movement. Eating without moving is like over-filling your car's gas tank without driving. The car won't take any more gas until you drive it, and your cells won't take more glucose if you're not moving.

There are lots of ways to get active, but most of us also face significant barriers to exercise. For one, many people with diabetes do not particularly enjoy vigorous exercise. Probably, this stems from a genetic tendency to conserve energy, and/or a long community history of working very, very hard and not having much to eat.

Yet people overcome their resistance and learn to enjoy exercise. In addition to reducing blood sugars, exercise has the following beneficial effects, all documented in studies:

- Improved mood, less depression.
- Better sleep.
- Less pain.
- Higher HDL ("good" cholesterol).
- More energy.
- Weight loss.
- Better bowel function.

It's a pretty good deal, and it doesn't cost much. The keys to success are:

Make it fun. Do something you enjoy. It might be playing a sport, or walking a dog, playing with children, dancing, water exercise, or some movement you happen to like. If you walk, walk somewhere pleasant or pretty. If you can't think of any pleasurable way to move, you may need to look for something new or ask for ideas.

Make it convenient. If you have to drive ten miles to the gym, you're going to stay home most times. The best exercises are the easiest: taking the stairs instead of the elevator, walking/ running in the neighborhood, stretching before you get out of bed. You can turn housework into a good workout or turn household items into weights for strengthening.

Make it social. Most people like exercise better if they do it with others. You can join a group or a gym, or just recruit a friend or family member to work out with. Perhaps you could start a group at your church or your job.

Make it comfortable. If you're walking, running or dancing, you'll need comfortable shoes that don't rub your feet. If you're riding a real bike or a stationary one, you can buy a comfortable seat, if the one it came with is too narrow.

Make it safe. Check your feet after walking or running to make sure there are no sores. You might want to apply a lotion afterward and massage the feet to improve circulation. When you increase your level of exercise, you should test your sugars before and after to see how much they come down. If you are on insulin or an insulin-stimulating drug, your sugars may get too low after exercise, unless you learn how much of a drop you can expect. You may need to cut your dose of these drugs as you work out more. Carry glucose gel or drops[21] with you for emergencies. Be aware that sugars can continue to drop for hours after exercise, as the muscles replenish their glucose supply. You may want to consult your doctor or diabetes educator for help with preventing low sugars. One other note: although exercise normally reduces glucose substantially, if your sugar is too high (say over 350) when you start, and you don't have enough circulating insulin, the glucose level may actually go up with exercise. Check with your doctor or educator if your sugars run that high.

Experiment. Everyone tells you to walk, but you might want to do other things. Strengthening is often more helpful than walking, because having more muscle will soak up glucose and decrease insulin resistance. So you might want to consider weight training. You don't necessarily have to join a gym. Leg lifts with heavy shoes, or arm lifts with heavy cans of food can strengthen you. Exercise also has emotional benefits, and aggressive forms of exercise may help you deal with anger and frustration. Consider a martial art like tai chi, karate or kickboxing.[7] Yoga is also a wonderful exercise. Water exercise puts less stress on legs and hips and can be enjoyable and relaxing. Generally, it's best to do more than one thing, so you don't get bored, and so more parts of you get involved.

Remember, the more physically active you are, the healthier you are likely to be, and the more you will be able to do for others. This is a dangerous time in the world, when we need the healthiest, most active people we can find. Start slow, build up, and see how far you can go.

What to Eat?

Healthy eating starts with attitude. Part of healthy eating is making peace with food, eating more slowly, enjoying it more. Worrying too much about what you eat is stressful. You don't want to be stressed while you're eating, because stress interferes with digestion. The controversy over the best diabetes diet also makes food choices more stressful. How do you know what to eat, and how can you consistently act on that knowledge?

I don't believe one diet is right for everyone. You need to find what works for you. You can do this by testing sugars after various foods and seeing how they affect your glucose levels.[8] You can use this information to avoid foods that make your sugars go up too much in the hours after eating. You might want to talk with a diabetes educator about the best ways to do this, if the books I suggest don't meet your needs. You won't have to do this forever. You work hard at the beginning learning about yourself; then things usually fall into place.

I'm going to suggest a general meal plan, based on Richard Bernstein and others. Feel free to ignore it if you want. There are many other sources of advice, including the books and web sites on the Resource List. First, it helps to understand the normal insulin response.

People without diabetes have stored insulin that jumps into the blood at the first sign of glucose. This is called the Phase 1 response, and allows non-diabetics to eat ice cream and cake without a spike in blood glucose level. People with T2D have little or no stored insulin, so no Phase 1. Eating stimulates your body to make more insulin, the Phase 2 response, but this takes time.

Most people with T2D still have a Phase 2 response. They make some insulin, so they can handle a certain amount of carbohydrates, if they're the kinds that turn into glucose slowly. This is why you want carbs with a low glycemic index (GI).[9] A low GI food turns into sugar slowly, so your Phase 2 response can still catch up to it. But you should not overeat even low GI foods, because your Phase 2 probably isn't that great. It would make sense to ask your doctor how much insulin you are still making. The more advanced your T2D is, the less insulin you are probably producing, and the more careful you have to be about carbs, especially if you're not injecting or inhaling insulin before meals.

If you follow the low-GI approach strictly, green, leafy vegetables are fine in T2D; eat all you want, within reason. Other non-starchy plant foods like green peppers, string beans and berries are good. Starchy fruits (like apples and pears) and starchy vegetables, truly whole grain breads and pastas are OK in small amounts, and refined carbohydrates not at all. Because of the addictive quality of refined flours and sugars, it may be easiest to avoid them completely. If you eat some, you'll want more and more.

It's good to get a glycemic index chart, because some foods will surprise you. Pizza, for example, raises a lot of people's blood sugars more rapidly than almost anything else. Even with a chart, you should still test yourself with various foods if you can. Everybody is different.

Protein is good. Your body will use some of it for construction and repair and break down the rest into glucose for fuel. This takes time, so your Phase 2 insulin response, if you have one, should have time to cover it. Fats never break down into glucose, and fatty acids can be used as energy, so unsaturated fats (like fish and nuts) are very good if you don't go crazy with them, and saturated fats (like beef, pork and cheese) OK in relatively small amounts.

In practice, this kind of eating is not so hard to do. It's similar to the South Beach diet[10] and the recommendations of programs like Food Addicts Anonymous. You basically eat large amounts of greens, either cooked or in salad form, along with protein at each meal. The salads can have small amounts of other fruits, nuts, animal or soy protein, or vegetables in them or on the side. Make sure you get some fat, primarily from fish or polyunsaturated oil a few times each day. You can find recipes for this kind of food in any low-carb cookbook or in magazines like *Diabetes Health*.[3]

This is the strict version. It's up to you how strict you want to be. If you simply stop or sharply limit refined flours and sugars (say by eating a salad with protein instead of a muffin in the morning), you will help yourself a lot.

The great advantage of this kind of eating plan is that you don't feel deprived. You're eating large quantities of green stuff, so you feel pretty full. Making it taste good is a bit of a challenge, but there are many seasonings and low-calorie dressings you can use, and so many potential ingredients to try, that most people find it surprisingly easy to stay with this plan. But there are some things to be aware of if you do:

- If you're on insulin or a sulfonylurea drug, you may need to lower the dose. Otherwise, you risk low blood sugar. Ask your doctor.
- Drink lots of water, because weight loss and high protein consumption create by-products that need to be diluted.
- If you're exercising a lot, you may need more carbs or fats for fuel.
- The total amount of calories you eat is important, too.
- This plan is great for losing weight. When you don't want to lose any more, you might need to slowly add more calories for energy.
- Never skip breakfast. You'll be grazing all day if you do. Always have some protein with breakfast (and most other meals).

Some other tips:
- It's much, MUCH easier to avoid temptation than to resist it. If you love cookies, don't bring them in the house. Don't

even walk down that aisle in the supermarket. You will need to negotiate some of this with your family. It's harder to avoid temptation at work and family events. The best you can do is make sure that you are not hungry when you go there. Eat before the event, make sure you have healthy snacks with you so you don't get hungry. Stay away from the candy bowl.

- Some people delight in getting you to eat more, so you need some assertiveness skills. Say Aunt Hilda offers me a big piece of homemade cake at a family party and implies she'll be really hurt if I don't eat it. If I am assertive, I can politely but firmly refuse. ("Thanks, Hilda. I don't want any cake now. Could I have a hug instead?")[11]
- This kind of eating may be more expensive, especially where vegetables are not readily available. This is where farmers' markets and food co-ops come into their own. Growing your own greens is also very cheap. If you want some saturated fat with your protein, you can save money and calories by using fast food's marketing strategy against them. Go in with a friend, order the super-size double burger, take off the bun, and split the meat. Bring your own bottles of (tap) water so you won't be tempted to buy a soda.
- Avoid prepared, packaged foods, especially things with high-fructose corn syrup and partially-hydrogenated oils ("trans-fats"). This is pretty much all packaged food. Learn to read labels.[12] Canned or frozen whole foods (like tuna or unsweetened fruit) can be OK, though.
- You'll probably need support to make these kinds of changes. Get some from friends, a support group, and other people with T2D or weight issues.[13]

The Power of Emotions

You'll be most vulnerable to unhealthy behaviors when dealing with hard emotions, like fear, depression, and anger. You want to find alternative ways to make yourself feel better. One idea is to give yourself a treat, such as a massage, hot shower, funny movie, or whatever works for you.

Hard lives and health problems bring up hard emotions, but they're there for a reason. If we work with them, they can help us make valuable changes. Grieving our losses helps us cope with them and helps us gain sympathy for ourselves and for others. Crying helps, and I keep records and videos around that I know make me cry for just this purpose. Laughter may be even better than sobbing, so comics or other things that make you laugh are good medicine.

Anger motivates change — use it to help you change a situation that is stressing you or your family. Anger also motivates exercise. Fear can be a great teacher, pointing us to what we need to change. If we don't face these emotions, we'll probably just treat them by eating. Get help with these issues from professionals, clergy, or friends.

Getting Centered

We know stress raises glucose and blood pressure, so stress reduction/management is crucial. Everyone should have something they do to relax them and to tune out the noise of daily living. These could include meditation, prayer, spending time in nature, listening to a guided imagery[14] or relaxation tape, playing music, or a dozen other things. Yoga and Tai chi combine relaxation with movement. Whatever works — the important thing is to do it regularly and not let all your other demands get in the way. If this means shutting a door or hiding under a bed, and screening your calls, do it.

These coping mechanisms may only take you so far, though. Sometimes you have to change stressful situations. This particularly applies to situations of work, relationships, and housing. Changing such things is usually more difficult than going for a walk or cutting out cookies. It often goes through many stages and involves getting help, but you can at least explore whether you can change a situation, change your response to it, or get out of it.

Listening to Your Body

In T2D, self-monitoring is the way to gain control. You can be a scientist, experimenting on yourself and recording the results. You will soon know more about how things like food, exercise, and stress affect you than your doctor or anyone else knows.

Unfortunately, glucose monitoring is often prescribed mindlessly. It doesn't do much good to stick yourself four times a day at the same times and worry about the results all night or not think about them again. You want to use testing to get information you can use. Don't test without a reason. Vary the times you check, and check when something new or interesting happens, a new food, a work responsibility, stressor, exercise program, or a new symptom. If all you're doing is keeping a log for your doctor, once a day is usually enough, just to protect against numbers creeping up. Having a regular A1C test is valuable to assess your overall control.

Testing is also an important safety measure against hypoglycemia when you're exercising a lot or going on a long drive, especially if you use insulin or a sulfonylurea drug. If you use insulin, testing can help you adjust your dose. Testing also protects against hyperglycemia when you're sick. Illness and infection tend to raise blood sugars, so you're likely to need to increase your medications and fluids and to call a doctor if sugars are too high.

Glucose checking can be a drag because of all the needle sticks. There will probably be no-stick ways of testing widely available soon, but for now, there are techniques to check your blood without much pain.[15]

Besides glucose testing, self-monitoring can also include:

- Your feet for any sign of skin breakdown or infection.
- Your blood pressure (BP). You can explore BP the same way you explore glucose levels, checking at different times or when different things happen. You may want to get your own blood pressure meter ("sphygmomanometer") to help.[16]
- Your energy level and mood — How good do you feel? You can rate energy and mood on a scale of 1–10.
- Your weight — Some people consider their weight the most important vital sign, but it's not. Glucose levels, blood pressure, and cholesterol are probably more important. But losing weight is still desirable if you're too heavy. Not all weight is the same, though. Abdominal fat tends to be bad for you, but fat in your lower half may be good. Muscle weighs more than fat, so getting stronger can increase your weight, but that is not a health problem. So waist size, (abdominal girth) is a better indicator of health than overall weight, but scale numbers do give you rapid feedback on how you're changing.

Self-monitoring is not the only monitoring. According to Dr. Steven Edelman, who lives with T1D and is author of *Taking Control of Your Diabetes,* you should see an ophthalmologist for your eyes once a year, see a podiatrist (foot doctor) and other specialists as needed, and have regular appointments with a doctor who can check your cholesterol, A1C, thyroid and kidney function, and support you in self-care.

This is a lot to keep track of. You don't need to do all of it all the time, but you should be as aware as you can be of what's happening. You can put it all in one log book[17] and bring it to your medical appointments. It's also useful to keep track of things in your life that might have affected your numbers. You and your medical team might learn a lot.

Do you have time to pay all this attention to your body? Do you want to? The answers to these questions will depend on how much you value yourself and how much support you've got. Frequently, we need to overcome some negative attitudes towards our bodies — ideas we picked up from the environment — if we want to give ourselves the attention we need and deserve. We need to get help with other demands to free up time for self-care.

Some people consider their weight or their blood glucose to be verdicts on how good they are as people. But a blood glucose level or a weight is not a judgment. It's a piece of experimental data, a scientific fact you can use to do better. Self-monitoring is not rocket science, but it is science, and you are the scientist, doing an ongoing investigation into yourself. It's not about good and bad; it's about learning and getting better at it.

How Tight Can You Go?

How tight should your glucose control be? ADA recommends shooting for an A1C of 7.0%. Most people with T2D run higher than that, but at 7.0%, you're still risking complications, since 7.0% corresponds to an average blood glucose of 147–172, far above normal. The American Association of Clinical Endocrinologists says 6.5% is better. Normal is 4.0–6.0%, and many diabetics do, in fact get under 6%. But others stay above 8% for years and never get complications.

So your goal is your call. The closer you get to 6.0%, the better you'll probably feel, and the less risk of complications you'll have. But tighter control means more work and a stricter food plan, and sometimes runs increased risk of hypoglycemic attacks. I think the tighter numbers are realistic and safe, but only if you stay on a very low glycemic index diet. Fast-acting carbs make your sugars go up, which raises your A1C, then crash down, risking hypoglycemia. On a low GI diet, you will be much safer from lows, so you can shoot for tighter control.

Medications

For all the bad things I said about drugs in Chapter 4, proper use of medications is important. Getting off medications is a realistic and desirable goal in T2D, but until you get there, medications can prevent a lot of damage. But there's a big trap to avoid. You start some new drug, your sugars go down somewhat, and you think you're managing your diabetes. So you don't make the life changes you need to make. A few years later, you're in trouble with complications. Drugs work better when they're part of a treatment plan that focuses on self-care.

But how do you know which ones are right for you? You can follow your doctor's orders unquestioningly, or you can participate in the decision. Doctors are experts in drugs, so their input is the first piece of information you need. But find out everything you can about any medication your doctor proposes — from websites, the doctor or other health workers, package inserts, people in your community, or support groups. Think about what benefits are promised and how good the evidence is that the drug actually works and is safe. Consider cost, side-effects, and the effort involved. Tell your doctor about your concerns — don't keep secrets to please him! You can use the same decision process for other potential therapies.

I have opinions about the value of various oral medications, but I'm not a doctor. If you're interested, e-mail me, and I'll send you some references.

The Insulin Question

Whether to take insulin is a big question people with T2D often face. Insulin used to be a late-stage treatment in T2D, and many people are scared of it, because they think going on insulin means they are dying or means their self-care has failed. But this isn't true anymore. More and more doctors are starting patients on insulin soon after diagnosis. The advantage is that insulin takes the load off beta cells and can keep glucose very close to normal, helping prevent complications. You might want to ask your doctor about starting on insulin if he or she doesn't suggest it.

The difficulty is that you need to test your sugars more to avoid lows, and maybe count carbs to know how much insulin to take. You may also gain weight if you don't adjust your food intake and exercise. However, you should be doing that anyway. The newer insulins are expensive, and the syringes and more frequent testing also cost money. Discuss all these issues with your doctor or diabetes educator before you start.

Having an insulin pump may be easiest; you won't need the shots because you're getting continuous insulin from the pump. The new inhaled insulins might be even better. You will need training on how to use any of the insulins.

Paying for drugs gets to be a big problem for a lot of people with T2D. If your health insurance doesn't cover your drugs, you can ask your doctor for cheaper or generic medicines. You can sometimes order larger doses and cut them in half to save money. You can sometimes get financial support from the manufacturers; most drug companies have such assistance programs.[18] The ADA gives good information on health insurance[19] and patient assistance programs.

Surgery is another option, but it changes your life in significant ways. You'll have to eat small amounts frequently for the rest of your life, and take a number of supplements to keep from malnutrition. But it works, and most people do well with it. If you're struggling, look into it. A couple of books on bariatric surgery are on the Resource List.[20]

Natural treatments

Nearly a dozen herbs have been shown in studies to lower blood sugars. These were small studies, often without a control group, so your doctor probably won't be telling you about them. And since there's little profit to be made, I wouldn't hold my breath waiting for better studies any time soon. But they may be worth trying. Here are six of them. Be aware that, if you are already taking other sugar-lowering medications, these might push your sugar too low, so you'll need to be careful when you start. Monitor your sugars after taking them and see what happens. You might need to lower or stop some medications.

Cinnamon. Just half a teaspoon of cinnamon a day significantly reduces blood sugar levels and LDL ("bad cholesterol"). Cinnamon oil doesn't work; you have to use the powdered kind. (*Diabetes Care,* vol 26, p 3125.)

Salacia. The Indian medicine Salacia oblonga seems to block the breakdown of carbs into glucose, and lowered post-meal glucose levels by 23%. (*Journal of the American Dietetic Association,* Feb 2005.)

Holy Basil (Ocimum sanctum). Holy Basil may improve beta cell function and insulin secretion. Holy basil is also used in India for arthritis, asthma, and heart problems. (*Diabetes Health,* September, 2005.)

Banaba (Lagerstroemia speciosa). 48 mg, given in a soft-gel capsule, lowered glucose by an average of 30%. These capsules are commercially available as a product called GlucoTrim. (*Journal of Pharmacological Sciences,* 93:69–73, 2003.)

(My thanks to Laura Shane McWhorter, PharmD, BC-ADM, CDE, writer for *Diabetes Health* for reporting some of this research.)

Other herbs that have shown themselves helpful in T2D include:

Gymnema. Indian scientists found in the 1990s that this herb may help repair damaged beta cells.

American ginseng (panax quinquefolius) seems to reduce after-meal glucose spikes.

Bitter melon, used in Chinese soups and other dishes, also has been found to lower blood sugars.

Risk Reduction

Healthy living is about more than sugar and weight control. **Smoking** and diabetes are a lethal combination, because they both damage blood vessels in similar ways. If you smoke more than a few cigarettes a day, stopping smoking is just as important as getting your glucose under control. Most doctors and communities have stop-smoking programs.

While small amounts of alcohol are probably OK in T2D, **excessive drinking** should be treated. For one thing, it makes other self-care behavior much more difficult.

Dental problems can really damage your glucose control. So frequent (preferably twice a day or more) flossing and brushing can make a big difference in your diabetes.

Avoid lows — Always carry some kind of glucose tabs or gels and have them handy at your bedside and in your car.[21] Don't skip meals, and test if you feel you are getting too low. Your medications might need to be adjusted downward as your lifestyle gets healthier.

Getting Help

Re-read Chapter 7. I always say that finding, asking for, and accepting help are the most important skills anyone with a long-term illness needs. This may involve unlearning a lot of bad ideas about independence and what constitutes strength.

Help can come from anywhere: family, friends, neighbors, other people with diabetes, your congregation (God is a reliable source of help for many people), people with shared interests, health care or other professionals, government or non-profit agencies, the American Diabetes Association, support groups[22] in-person or on the Internet, even pets. You just have to be willing to ask and accept. Isolation and diabetes are a bad combination. If being social has always been a problem for you, you might get some professional help with that.

You really want to get help from your medical team. You can help them help you in several ways.

- Prepare for appointments — know what you want and bring a written list of questions and concerns. Bring records of your self-monitoring results and recent visits to other providers. Bring your medications and some way to record the appointment — a notebook or a tape recorder if that's OK with the staff.
- Bring a friend or family member with you as an extra pair of ears, eyes, and lips.
- Relate to the doctor and other staff as people, and try to let them know who you are as a person. If they're not willing or able to form a relationship, you may want to look for somebody else.
- Ask about group appointments, support groups, or other ways the system can hook you up with other patients. Perhaps they have a social worker who can connect you with resources in the community, say help with food, a free place to work out or socialize.

Getting your family on board is even more crucial. How can you keep cookies out of your sight if everyone else wants them? Behavior change challenges families to communicate better and resolve problems. Remember that healthy diabetes living is healthier for everyone. When one person in a family has T2D, others are at risk, so try to make health a family affair.

Some more general tips on getting help:

- Don't get all your help in one place, as some people do with their spouse or partner. You'll burn the helper out and miss out on other, more effective sources. No one person is good at everything. Have a team.
- Be specific. Don't make vague requests, or people will be afraid they're making a lifetime commitment. If your request is specific, they'll know what they're getting into.

- Don't apologize. People don't want to know how much your feet hurt or what your latest EKG showed. Just say, "Please, could you help me with X?
- It's easy to repay people — with thanks, by listening to them, by doing something for them or for others less fortunate ("pay it forward").

Reasons to Live

Here's a prediction. You won't do any of this stuff if you don't have a good reason to. We all need reasons to live — sources of meaning, purpose, pleasure, love, growth, and fun. Your reasons don't have to be important to anyone except you, but quite probably, when you give attention and energy to your reasons to live, you will make the people around you feel better, too.

Reasons to live often involve helping other people. This can mean volunteering somewhere, working in a job that involves helping others, or just caring for the people around you. Building the wellness movement by helping others to take care of themselves, or improving the environment for your family or community are great reasons to live.

There's one way to help that any of us can do, at any state of health or ability. By doing our best, by not giving up, we become an inspiration to others. We may not like it, but it goes with the territory, and it has value. We have a saying in MS support groups — "One person coping helps everyone cope." Sounds like a greeting card, doesn't it? But it's so true, and it's so powerful. If you can just keep showing up at work or in the community or at support group with a positive, caring attitude, you will help everyone else keep going.

One person coping with diabetes can help a whole family or a whole neighborhood cope. A parent coping with diabetes can help children and grandchildren avoid getting it. So when you take care of yourself, you're not just doing it for you. A lot of other people are pulling for you, and a lot of other people will benefit from your success. I hope you go beyond self-care and help change the political and social environment, but if you're taking care of yourself, you're part of the movement. Welcome.

Appendix B

Resource List

I'M SORRY THAT A LOT of these resources are web sites. If you don't have home access, I hope your local library or Internet café, or a friend or relative can get you on-line.

1. Write me at Nurse@davidsperorn.com or visit www.art-of-getting-well.com.
2. Some good all-around general information books are:

American Diabetes Association. *ADA Complete Guide to Diabetes: The Ultimate Home Diabetes Reference from the Diabetes Experts.* Bantam, 1997. Their dietary advice, however, is too rich in carbohydrates, according to the other resources listed here.

Bernstein, Richard. *Dr. Bernstein's Diabetes Solution: The Complete Guide to Achieving Normal Blood Sugars, Revised Edition.* Little, Brown, 2003.

Becker, Gretchen. *Type 2 Diabetes: The First Year — An Essential Guide for the Newly Diagnosed.* Constable & Robinson Ltd, 2004.

Some good books on self-management are:

Spero, David, RN. *The Art of Getting Well: Maximizing Health When You Have a Chronic Illness.* Hunter House, 2002.

Polonsky, William. *Diabetes Burnout: Preventing It, Surviving It, Finding Inner Peace.* ADA, 1999.

Holman, Halsted, David Sobel, Virginia Gonzalez, Diana Laurent, Marian Minor, and Kate Lorig. *Living a Healthy Life with Chronic Conditions.* Publishers Group West, 2000.

On the psychological and spiritual sides of living with diabetes:

Rubin, Richard, June Biermann, and Barbara Toohey. *Psyching Out Diabetes: A Positive Approach to Your Negative Emotions.* McGraw Hill, 1999.

Feste, Catherine. *Meditations on Diabetes: Strengthening Your Spirit in Every Season.* ADA, 1999.

3. Web MD's site webmd.com/diseases_and_conditions/diabetes.htm is good, although, again, their diet advice is similar to ADA's, which means awfully generous with the carbs.

Diabetes Self-Management magazine and diabetesselfmanagement.com/. Or call 800-234-0923 for a subscription.

Diabetes in Control, a free weekly newsletter, is geared more towards professionals, but a lot of others may find it informative. It advocates for the low-carb approach. diabetesincontrol.com/index.php.

Diabetes Health magazine and website is a wealth of practical information and good stories. Joy Pape's diet, recipe and support column is particularly worth checking out. On-line at diabeteshealth.com/ or for a subscription call 800-488-8468.

Diabetes Forecast, about living with diabetes, and new trends in treatment and research, is available from the ADA at diabetes.org/diabetes-forecast.jsp.

4. You can find a diabetes educator near you by calling American Association of Diabetes Educators at 800-338-3633.

5. For more on AADE 7, contact Milner-Fenwick at 1-800-432-8433 for a good video on diabetes self-management for about $15.

6. See listing in the Health Providers section of this list for self-management programs.

7. Find out more about tai chi, including where to find a tai chi instructor specifically for diabetes at Dr. Paul Lam's site www.taichifordiabetes.com.

   For an overview of martial arts in diabetes visit Diabetes Health Connection at diabeteshealthconnection.com/healthy_living/staying_in_shape/cardio_activities/article_12374.aspx.

8. An excellent guide to glucose testing is in Dr. Bernstein's *Diabetes Solution:* p. 73–89.

9. A thorough explanation of glycemic index is available at www.mendosa.com/gi.htm with an accompanying list of the GI of 750 foods at www.mendosa.com/gilists.htm.

10. Agatston, Arthur. *The South Beach Diet : The Delicious, Doctor-Designed, Foolproof Plan for Fast and Healthy Weight Loss.* St. Martin's Griffin, 2003.

11. A strong on-line assertiveness training class can be found at mentalhelp.net/psyhelp/chap13/chap13e.htm.

    Classes in assertiveness and communication skills are also available at many medical centers and community centers.

12. A good explanation of food labels is given by the ADA at diabetes.org/nutrition-and-recipes/nutrition/foodlabel.jsp.

13. Food Addicts Anonymous is a 12-step program that provides social support and a strict diet plan. Visit foodaddictsanonymous.org.

    Weight Watchers also provides social support, but its focus is more on losing weight, not diabetes or wellness.

    Overeaters Anonymous, another 12-step recovery program, provides social support without any diet recommendations or rules. They have telephone and on-line meetings as well as face-to-face gatherings. oa.org

14. My favorite guided imagery books and tapes are Martin Rossman's, including *Guided Imagery for Self-Healing: An Essential Resource for Anyone Seeking Wellness*. H. J. Kramer, 2000. Tapes are available at academyforguidedimagery .com/selfhealing.php.
    Also Belleruth Naparstek's tapes at healthjourneys.com

15. Less-painful glucose testing ideas in Dr. Bernstein's *Diabetes Solution*, p 77.

16. The American Association of Family Practitioners advocates home blood pressure monitoring at familydoctor .org/128.xml, including information on what equipment you might want to get. Alternatively, your local medical center or pharmacy might offer blood pressure checks in your community.

17. There are hundreds of diabetes logs and diaries available to buy, or you can make your own. An example is at diabetes managementworks.ca/.

18. A listing of drug company patient assistance programs can be found at needymeds.com, or you can call the drug manufacturer directly.

19. ADA information on health insurance can be found at diabetes.org/advocacy-and-legalresources/healthcare/insurance.jsp, or call 1-800-DIABETES.

20. Learn more about bariatric surgery pros and cons at http://win.niddk.nih.gov/publications/gastric.htm.
    A book that takes a skeptical view of bariatric surgery is Fox, S. Ross, MD's. *The Patient's Guide to Weight Loss Surgery: Everything You Need To Know About Gastric Bypass and Bariatric Surgery*. Hatherleigh Press, 2004.
    A book more favorable to surgery and probably a more helpful assessment is Paula Peck's *Exodus from Obesity: The Guide to Long-Term Success After Weight Loss Surgery*, BP Publishing, 2003.

21. If you are on insulin or a sulfonylurea, it is important to

carry some glucose gel or tablets with you with you at all times. Call Diabetic Express at 1-800-338-4656 or find other sources and information on treating low blood sugars at mendosa.com/hypoglycemic_supplies.htm.

22. Support groups are extremely valuable. Your medical team may be able to provide you with a list of them in your community. The Diabetes Association is another good resource for support groups. Call them at 1-800-DIABETES. The Diabetes Information Center website has a list of support groups for all 50 states: elviradarknight.com/diabetes/ supportgroups.html. So does defeatdiabetes.org/support_groups.htm.

Outside the USA, there are fewer support groups, but the Internet support groups are great if you're far away from a group. Web MD has a good group at boards.webmd .com/topic.asp?topic_id=1011. On-line diabetes chats are happening at diabetic-talk.org.

Resources for Communities

- 100 Black Men: 100blackmenba.org/youthmovement.htm
- Health Conductors: babuf.org/ or call Colette Winlock 510-763-7270.
- Project Dulce, a collaboration of health care and community-based organizations, universities, clinics and promotores: 1-866-791-8154 or e-mail Anna Garay garay.anna@scripps health.org.
- Regional Center for Border Health, information on extensive health promotion and healthcare programs: snap211.com/org/1921134.html.
- Latino Health Access — diabetes training, community organizing, and promotores training: 1717 N Broadway Santa Ana, CA 92706, 714-542-7792, latinohealthaccess .org/index.shtml.
- Find out more about community health workers at the

Massachusetts Community Health Worker Network: contact Lisa Renee Siciliano, MACHW at 508-791-5893 or email Lrsiciliano@aol.com.

- Food co-ops — Local Harvest Food Co-op's site includes listings of hundreds of existing co-ops: localharvest.org/food-coops/. There are also Community Supported Agriculture (CSA) farms, where communities can subscribe directly with farmers and receive regular shipments of produce: csacenter.org/.
- The National Association of Farmers' Markets in England: PO Box 575, Southampton, SO15 7BZ Tel: 0845 45 88.
- A listing of many farmers' markets in the US is at cafecreo sote.com/Farmers_Markets/.
- Vancouver's City Farmer organization, an informational gold mine for those interested in urban farming, 604-736-2250 or visit their website at cityfarmer.org/.
- The Food and Agriculture Organization of the United Nations promotes urban agriculture. Contact George Kourous, Information Officer, FAO by email george.kourous@fao.org or call (+39) 06 570 53168.
- Nurse Family Partnership — You may well be able to bring this program to your area: nursefamilypartnership.org/index.cfm?fuseaction=home or write 1900 Grant Street, Suite 400, Denver, CO 80203 or call 866-864-5226 or e-mail info@nursefamilypartnership.org.
- CATCH Program, Texas office: sph.uth.tmc.edu/chppr/catch/.
- Sports, Play, and Active Recreation for Kids: at sparkpe.org/.

Resources for Health Care Providers

- A center for self-management training is Stanford Patient Education Research Center, the original source for self-management training: at 650-723-4000 or http://patienteducation.stanford.edu. But many other sources offer it.

- Experts on patient empowerment are at: Michigan Diabetes Research and Training Center, 1331 E. Ann St., Box 0560, Room 5111, Ann Arbor, MI 48109-0580 or call 734-763-5730.
- If you're considering group appointments (and you should), look at the "Starter Kit" provided by Improving Chronic Illness Care (ICIC) improvingchroniccare.org/improvement /docs/startkit.doc, or call 206-287-2704.
- For resources on Self-Management Support: contact ICIC at improvingchroniccare.org.
- Find studies and programs on community supports for diabetes management at diabetesnpo.im.wustl.edu.
- Funding and new programs: The Institute for Healthcare Improvement is reforming health care from the inside: ihi.org.
- Robert Wood Johnson Foundation, the biggest funder of research on SMS programs and many social approaches to health in the US: rwjf.org/index.jsp.
- The Canadian Institutes of Health Research (CIHR) has funded research on SMS: mcmaster.ca/ors/sources/cihr /cihr_intro.htm.

Fighting for Universal Coverage

- An organization called Results is organizing for health care coverage for all by 2010, in line with the recommendation of the Institute of Medicine. Visit results.org/website/article .asp?id=1459.
- Other groups working on this include Health Care Now, 339 Lafayette Street, New York, NY 10012. Call 212-475-8350, e-mail info@healthcare-now.org, and the The Women's Universal Health Initiative, 190 Alleghany Street, Boston, MA 02120. Contact Catherine DeLorey, Coordinator, at cdelorey@earthlink.net, or call 617-739-2923.

- Citizens' Health Care Working Group was created by the federal government, but seems to be serious about getting people involved. Go to citizenshealthcare.gov/ to participate directly.

Notes

Introduction

1. Rosen, George, "The Evolution of Social Medicine," in Freeman, Howard, S. Levine, L. Reeder, eds. *Handbook of Medical Sociology*, Rosen, George Prentice-Hall, 1972.

Prologue

1. On the basic physiology of diabetes American Diabetes Association. *ADA Complete Guide to Diabetes: The Ultimate Home Diabetes Reference.* Bantam, 1997.

    Bernstein, Richard. *Dr. Bernstein's Diabetes Solution: The Complete Guide to Achieving Normal Blood Sugars, Revised Edition.* Little, Brown, 2003.
2. Moller, David E. *Insulin Resistance.* John Wiley & Sons, 1993.
3. Diabetes Statistics from National Diabetes Information Clearinghouse "National Diabetes Statistics," http://diabetes.niddk.nih.gov/dm/pubs/statistics, site accessed January 3, 2006.

4. The costs are probably underestimated. Government reports say the average annual medical expenses are about $13,000 per person with diabetes, as compared to $2,500 for the average person without diabetes. Multiply the $10,500 difference by the 20 million people with diabetes, and you get $210 billion in medical expenses alone. The discrepancy seems to come from the fact that many diabetes complication-related expenses are counted as kidney disease or heart disease or other medical expenses, instead of as diabetes.

5. Bowman, Lee. "Most people with diabetes fail to control blood sugar," Scripps Howard News Service, May 19, 2005.

6. American Diabetes Association, "Diabetes Epidemic Grows as Feds Reduce Commitment to Prevention," statement published in *Diabetes in Control,* December 27, 2005. diabetesincontrol.com/modules.php?name=News&file=article&sid=3370, site accessed January 10, 2006.

7. McFarlane Samy, R. L. Chaiken, S. Hirsch, P. Harrington, H. E. Lebovitz, M. A. Banerji. "Near-normoglycaemic remission in African-Americans with Type 2 diabetes mellitus is associated with recovery of beta cell function." *Diabetes Medicine,* 18(1):10–6, January 2001.

8. Orchard, Trevor, M. Temprosa, R. Goldberg, S. Haffner, R. Ratner, S. Marcovina, S. Fowler, "The effect of metformin and intensive lifestyle intervention on the metabolic syndrome: the Diabetes Prevention Program randomized trial." *Annals of Internal Medicine.* 142(8):611–9, April 2005.

9. Information on the history of arthritis from www.pehp.org/phc/healthtracks/pdf/section3/arthritis.pdf, site visited January 2006.

10. Historical information about diabetes from: Ekoe, Jean-Marie. *Diabetes Mellitus: Aspects of the World-wide Epidemiology of Diabetes Mellitus and Its Long-Term Complications.* John Wiley & Sons, 2001.

11. Charles, R. W., and F. Medard. "Relation of diabetes to nutrition in Haiti," *Diabetes Abstracts,* 18 (Supp 1): 349, 1969.

Chapter 1

1. Numerous sources, all of which give slightly different estimates, include "National Diabetes Statistics" National Diabetes Information Clearinghouse http://diabetes.niddk.nih .gov/dm/pubs/statistics, site accessed January 2006.

Songer, Thomas Ph.D., Lorraine Ettaro, BSc and the Economics of Diabetes Project Panel. "Studies on the Cost of Diabetes," Centers for Disease Control and Prevention, National Center for Chronic Disease Prevention and Health Promotion, cdc.gov/diabetes/pubs/costs, site accessed January 2006.

I refer to these documents several times in this chapter.

2. "Either you're doing something wrong or..." A good example of blaming the victim, or the victim's genes is: Duenwald, Mary. "Diabetes: Faces of an Epidemic: From Mother to Daughter, Shared Genes and a Burden," *New York Times,* June 6, 2004.

Duenwald writes, "Type 2 diabetes has genetic foundations...the disease is prevalent in certain ethnic groups: Hispanics, African-Americans, American Indians, Alaska Natives, Asian-Americans and Pacific Islanders." Note the unsupported jump from "higher prevalence" to "genetic foundations." Is everyone but Europeans genetically damaged? How could this be?

An academic example of this is: Williams, R. C., J. C. Long, R. L. Hanson, M. L. Sievers, W. C. Knowler. "Individual estimates of European genetic admixture associated with lower body-mass index, plasma glucose, and prevalence of type 2 diabetes in Pima Indians," *American Journal of Genetics,* 66(2), February 2000. These learned scholars found that having more European ancestry correlated with fewer cases of diabetes, and conclude that genes must be responsible. Discrimination, poverty and job status were not controlled for.

3. *Diabetes in America, 2nd Edition,* National Diabetes Information Clearing House, National Institute of Diabetes, Digestive and Kidney Diseases, diabetes.niddk.nih.gov/dm/pubs /america, site accessed January 2006.

Diabetes Atlas, 2nd Edition, International Diabetes Federation, available from IDF www.idf.org, site accessed January 2006.

4. Read more about the fascinating science of epigenetics (how genes and environments interact) in: Ridley, Matt. *Nature Via Nurture: Genes, Experience and What Makes Us Human,* Harper Collins, 2003.

5. Talk by Indian Health Service doctor Adriann Begay, M.D. American Medical Association December 2003 Interim Meeting ama-assn.org/ama1/pub/upload/mm/20/drbegay dec2003.pdf, site accessed January 2006.

6. "Pima in Mexico have no more diabetes than their non-Pima neighbors..." And their genes apparently aren't much different either. They all gain weight when they're physically inactive. See: Fox, C.S., et al. "Is a low leptin concentration, a low resting metabolic rate, or both the expression of the 'thrifty genotype'? Results from Mexican Pima Indians," *American Journal of Clinical Nutrition,* 68(5):1053–7, November 1998.

7. Ratner, David, Ph.D. "The River People," *Psychology Today,* July 2002. psychologytoday.com/articles/pto-20020802-0 00029.html, site accessed January 13, 2006.

8. *Diabetes in America, 2nd Edition* gives diabetes statistics for all ages, classes, racial groups and geographic areas. These clearly show the relation between power and diabetes. The proportion of Type 2 diabetics who have completed at least some college education is 21.0% as compared to 40.3%

among those without diabetes. 15.6% of people with Type 2 diabetes have a family income > $40,000, compared to 32.8% of non-diabetic persons. The proportion of people with family income < $10,000 is 27.9% in T2D, and 12.6% in non-diabetic persons At every age, persons with Type 2 diabetes are less likely to be employed. In 1989, 66.2% of non-diabetic persons were employed, compared to 32.7% of people with Type 2 diabetes. People with Type 2 diabetes are much more likely than non-diabetics to be military veterans.

Government estimates are that 20% of Native Americans, about 15% of African-Americans and Latinos and 8.5% of non-Hispanic whites above the age of 20 have T2D. Many experts believe the actual numbers are far higher.

In 1995, 58.2% of Type 2s were women, significantly higher than the 52.4% of the general population who are women. Of Native Americans aged 45–74, 40% to 70% had diabetes in a recent screening in Arizona, Oklahoma, and the Dakotas. People of color, especially Blacks, American Indians and Hispanics, also have much higher rates of diabetes complications. See: Lee, Elisa. "Diabetes and impaired glucose tolerance in three American Indian populations aged 45–74 years," *Diabetes Care,* 18(5), 599–610, 1995.

9. "The same is true for individuals..." These statistics can be found at *Diabetes in America,* but many other studies confirm them. One example is: Brunner, Eric, M. J. Shipley, D. Blane, G. Davey Smith and M. G. Marmot. "Past and present socioeconomic circumstances and cardiovascular risk factors in adulthood," *Journal of Epidemiology and Community Health,* 53:757–764, 1999.

In fact, socioeconomic status (SES) is the single best predictor of chronic illness next to age. See also: Marmot, Michael. "Social Class, Occupational Status and Coronary Vascular Disease," *Occupational Medicine,* 15(1), 2000.

10. "Trauma can rob you of power..." There are many studies on this. In Chapter 2, I outline how trauma can increase stress levels for years, maybe for the rest of your life. See: Weisberg, Risa, S. E. Bruce, J. T. Machan, R. C. Kessler, L. Culpepper, M. B. Keller. "Non-psychiatric illness among primary care patients with trauma histories and posttraumatic stress disorder," *Psychiatric Services,* 53(7):848–54, July 2002.

Creighton, Susan J. "Child Abuse Trends in England and Wales," National Society for the Prevention of Cruelty to Children London, 1992.

Williamson, David, T. J. Thompson, R. F. Anda, W. H. Dietz, and V. Felitti. "Body weight and obesity in adults and self-reported abuse in childhood," *International Journal of Obesity and Related Metabolic Disorders,* 26(8):1075–82, August 2002.

Romans, Sarah, C. Belaise, J. Martin, E. Morris, and A. Raffi. "Childhood abuse and later medical disorders in women: an epidemiological study," *Psychotherapeutics and Psychosomatics,* 71(3):141–50, May/June 2002.

11. "Insecure home or [troubled] parents..." As I'll keep coming back to, most illness starts in childhood, if not before. Good studies include: Lundberg, Olle. "The impact of childhood living conditions on illness and mortality in adulthood," in *Social Science and Medicine,* 36 1047, 1993.

Felitti, Vincent J., et al. "Relationship of childhood abuse and household dysfunction to many of the leading causes of death in adults: The Adverse Childhood Experiences (ACE) Study," *American Journal of Preventive Medicine,* 14(4):245–58, May 1998. Dr. Felitti has performed dozens of powerful studies linking tough childhoods to almost every conceivable health problem.

12. Why this is hasn't been studied, but Veteran Affairs is well aware of it. More than one in six VA patients have T2D. You

would think that with the ever-increasing number of veterans in America, someone would wonder why so many vets are so sick. See *Diabetes in America, 2ⁿᵈ Edition* and va.gov/health/diabetes/default.htm, site accessed January 2006.

13. I thank Ane McDonald, a brilliant Native American researcher for alerting the world to this amazing situation.

McDonald, Ane. "Diabetes in Two Cuahuilla Indian Communities: A Case Study of the Riverside-San Bernardino Indian Health Diabetes Program and Two of the Communities it Serves," in Samuels & Associates, "The Social & Environmental Experience of Diabetes, a Series of Case Studies," Prepared for the California Endowment, 2003.

14. Maté, Gabor. *When The Body Says No,* John Wiley & Sons, 2003.

15. "Tuberculosis used to be considered an inherited weakness..." Dormandy, Thomas. *The White Death: A History of Tuberculosis,* New York University Press, 2000.

16. Lantz, Paula, J. S. House, J. M. Lepkowski, D. R. Willams, R. P. Mero, and J. Chan. "Socioeconomic Factors, Health Behaviors, and Mortality," *Journal of the American Medical Association,* 279 (21) 1703–1708, June 3 1998.

17. Lantz, Paula, J. W. Lynch, J. S. House, J. M. Lepkowski, R. P. Mero, M. A. Musick, and D. R. Williams. "Socioeconomic disparities in health change in a longitudinal study of US adults: the role of health-risk behaviors," *Social Science and Medicine,* 53(1):29–40, July 2001.

18. Curves gyms have been strongly criticized for two things—the owner's support of anti-abortion activism and the low level of their workouts. But, despite these criticisms, I think they're better than nothing, and many women have started on a path toward healthier living there. Hopefully better services are available where you live, or soon will be.

Chapter 2

1. Sapolsky, Robert. *Why Zebras Don't Get Ulcers,* W. H. Freeman, 1994. This is by far the best book on stress and its physical and emotional effects, and one of the best pop science books I've ever read. It's easy to understand, entertaining and well documented. See also: Brandi, L. S., D. Santoro, A. Natali, F. Altomonte, S. Baldi, S. Frascerra, and E. Ferranini. "Insulin resistance of stress: sites and mechanisms," *Clinical Science,* 85 (525), 1993.

2. Talbott, Shawn. *The Cortisol Connection: Why Stress Makes You Fat and Ruins Your Health, And What You Can Do About It.* Hunter House Publishers, 2002. This book has very good explanations of how stress can lead to overweight.

3. "Repair can wait until the crisis is over..." Stress expert Bruce McEwen calls this "allostatic load," the process by which stress leads to illness. See his book, *The End of Stress as We Know It,* National Academies Press, 2002. Sapolsky's book also has good information on this.

4. Cox, Daniel, and Linda Gonder-Frederick. "The Role of Stress in Diabetes Mellitus." in McCabe, Philip, Neil Schneiderman, Tiffany Field, and Jay Skyler, eds. *Notes on Stress, Coping, and Disease,* Lawrence Earlbaum and Associates, 1991.

5. "Racism, sexism..." see: Tull, Eugene S., Y. T. Sheu, C. Butler, and K. Cornelious. "Relationships between perceived stress, coping behavior and cortisol secretion in women with high and low levels of internalized racism," *Journal of the National Med Association,* 97(2):206–12, February 2005. McEwan and Sapolsky also address this relationship.

6. "British studies proved that lower SES..." See any of Michael Marmot's studies starting with Whitehall I, many of which are described in Wilkinson, Richard, and Michael

Marmot. *Social Determinants of Health,* Oxford University Press 1999.

7. Lynch, James J. *The Language of the Heart.* Basic Books, 1986. Pickering T. "'White-coat hypertension:' should it be treated or not?" *Cleveland Clinic Journal of Medicine,* 69(8):584–5, August 2002.

8. "Hypertension is often a warning of coming diabetes..." Hypertension doesn't necessarily cause diabetes, but the two are frequently seen together. They are two elements of the so-called "metabolic syndrome" or "Syndrome X." (The other elements are high levels of bad cholesterols and over-weight, especially abdominal fat. Stress and depression are also frequent corollaries of metabolic syndrome.)

9. Gilbert, Paul. Depression: The Evolution of Powerlessness, Guilford Publications, 1992.

Gilbert, Paul. *Overcoming Depression, 2nd Edition.* Oxford University Press, 2001.

It's amazing what you can learn from the animals. Both of these books are based on animal studies. For human studies see: Trower, Peter, and Paul Gilbert. "Evolution and Process in Social Anxiety," in Crozier, W. Ray, and Lynn Alden, eds. *International Handbook of Social Anxiety: Concepts, Research and Interventions Relating to the Self and Shyness.* John Wiley & Sons, 2001.

10. Wilkinson, Richard. *Unhealthy Societies.* Routledge, 1997.

11. Statistics on Cuban vs. American life span and health spending are from: *Health Care Spending, UC Atlas of Global Inequality,* available at ucatlas.ucsc.edu/spend.php. The latest (2004) figures are 76.1 years of age in the US and 75.2 years of age in Cuba. Spending equals $4,500 per capita in the US, $220 per capita in Cuba.

12. Sapolsky, Robert. "Poverty's Remains," *The Sciences,* 31:8–10, 1991.

13. "biggest risk factors for abuse are marital problems,

unemployment, and debt..." Creighton, S. J. *Child Abuse Trends in England and Wales.* National Society for Prevention of Cruelty to Children London, 1992.

14. Francis, Darlene, Josie Diorio, Liu Dong, and Michael J. Meaney. "Non-genomic Transmission Across Generations of Maternal Behavior and Stress Responses in the Rat," *Science,* 286(5442):1155–1158, November 5 1999. There are dozens of studies on the same topic performed on primates.

15. Pryce, Christopher, A. C. Dettling, M. Spengler, C. R. Schnell, and J. Feldon. "Deprivation of parenting disrupts development of homeostatic and reward systems in marmoset monkey offspring," *Biological Psychiatry,* 15:56(2):72–9, July 2004.

16. Pryce, Christopher, Daniela Rüedi-Bettschen, Andrea Dettling, and Joram Feldon. "Early Life Stress: Long-Term Physiological Impact in Rodents and Primates," *News Physiol Sci,* 17: 150–155, 2002.

17. Meaney, M. J., M. Szyf. "Environmental programming of stress responses through DNA methylation: life at the interface between a dynamic environment and a fixed genome," *Dialogues in Clinical Neuroscience,* 7(2):103–23, 2005.

18. Elias, Marilyn. "Americans with major depression don't get adequate treatment," *Disability Employment News,* June 19, 2003.

19. Boscarino, J.A. "Post-traumatic stress disorder and physical illness: results from clinical and epidemiologic studies," *Annals of New York Academy of Science,* 1032:141–53, December 2004.

20. For more information on Cherokee history and the Trail of Tears see: Cherokee.org/Culture?historyPage.asp?Id=128, site accessed January 2006.

21. Lynch, Karen. "Native People Work to Heal Bitter Legacy of Government Boarding Schools," *Lakota Journal.* June 26, 2004.

22. Scannapieco, F.A. "Systemic effects of periodontal diseases," *Dent Clin North Am,* 49(3):533–50, vi., July 2005.
Sedano, Heddie O., DDS. "Dental Implications of Diabetes Mellitus," dent.ucla.edu/ftp/pic/visitors/Diabetes/incidence, site accessed January 2006.

23. Michalek, J. E., N. S. Ketchum, and R. C. Tripathi. "Diabetes mellitus and 2,3,7,8-tetrachlorodibenzo-p-dioxin elimination in veterans of Operation Ranch Hand," *Journal of Toxicology and Environmental Health,* 66(3):211–21, February 14, 2003.

24. Lockwood, Alan M.D. "Diabetes and Air Pollution," *Diabetes Care* 25:1487–1488, 2002

Chapter 3

1. Schlosser, Eric. *Fast Food Nation,* Houghton Mifflin Company, 2001. Chapter 6 discusses feedlots in depth. For purposes of this discussion, I'm not saying feedlots for cattle are inherently bad, but the cattle are not healthy and require a variety of medicines to keep them from getting sick. Humans who live like cattle are likely to do worse.
See eatwild.com/references.html#antibiotics, site accessed January 2006.

2. Critser, Greg. *Fatland: How Americans Became the Fattest People On Earth,* Houghton Mifflin Company, 2003. This is a particularly good resource for the history of HFCS, palm oil and the surplus of sugars, fats and refined carbohydrates in North American foods.

3. Two good books on the food industry and their political clout are:
Brownell, Kelly, and Katherine Battle Horgen. *Food Fight,* McGraw-Hill, 2004.
Nestle, Marion. *Food Politics: How the Food Industry Influences Nutrition and Health,* University of California, 2002.

4. Brownell, Kelly, Ph.D., and Marion Nestle, Ph.D. "The

Sweet and Lowdown on Sugar," *New York Times,* January 23, 2004.

5. A sample of these laws protecting industry:

Barnes, Tom. "Food industry blocking lawsuits over obesity," *Pittsburgh Post-Gazette,* April 19, 2005.

"Senate passes bill banning obesity-related lawsuits," *Las Vegas Review-Journal,* April 23, 2005.

"Obesity lawsuit ban passes U.S. House of Reps," pizza marketplace.com, March 11, 2004.

"Obesity Lawsuit Bill Protects State Restaurants," *Detroit News,* October 11, 2004.

6. Petersen, Melody. "Breastfeeding Ads Delayed By a Dispute Over Content," *New York Times,* December 4, 2003.

7. Brownell, Chapter 7.

8. Borwoski, John. "Caffeine and the First Amendement," counterpunch.com/borowski1231.html, site accessed January 2006.

9. Bovard, James. " Archer Daniels Midland: A Case Study In Corporate Welfare," cato.org/pubs/pas/pa-241.html, site accessed January 2006.

10. Morland, K., S. Wing, and C. Poole. "The contextual effect of the local food environment on residents' diets," *American Journal of Public Health,* 92:1761–1787, 2002.

11. Peacock, Elaine. "Mobilizing Local Resources and Informal Systems," in Samuels and Associates. *The Social and Environmental Experience of Diabetes: A Series of Case Studies,* California Endowment, 2003.

12. Poulter, S., and B. Hale. "Poor families priced out of a healthy diet," *Daily Mail,* October 24, 2001 (cited in Brownell p. 208).

13. Brownell, p. 210–213.

14. Des Maisons, Kathleen. *Potatoes not Prozac,* Simon and Schuster, 1998.

15. Cheraskin, E., M.D., and W. M. Ringsdorf, DMD. "A

biochemical denominator in the primary prevention of alcoholism," *Journal of Orthomolecular Psychiatry,* 9(3):158–163, 1980.

16. Colantuoni, C., et al. "Excessive sugar intake alters binding to dopamine and mu-opioid receptors in the brain," *NeuroReport,* 12:3549–3552, 2001.

And "Evidence that intermittent, excessive sugar intake causes endogenous opioid dependence," *Obesity Research,* 20:478–488, 2002.

17. Wurtman, R. J., and J. J. Wurtman. "Brain serotonin, carbohydrate-craving, obesity and depression," *Obesity Research,* 3 Suppl 4:477S–480S, November 1995.

18. Drenowski, A., D. D. Krahn, M. A. Demitrack, K. Nairn, and B. A. Gosnell. "Naloxone, an opiate blocker, reduces the consumption of sweet high-fat foods in obese and lean female binge eaters," *American Journal of Clinical Nutrition,* 61:1206–1212, 1995.

19. "Sugar in another form…" This is usually called the Glycemic Index (GI). A food's GI is the rate at which it breaks down into sugar. Many white breads and refined carbohydrates actually put glucose into the blood faster than some sugars. Many of my overweight interview subjects told me, "I don't like sugars, but I can't keep away from that bread." See: Brand-Miller, Jennie, Thomas Wolever, Kaye Foster-Powell, and Stephen Colagiuri. *The New Glucose Revolution: The Authoritative Guide to the Glycemic Index — the Dietary Solution for Lifelong Health,* Marlowe & Company, 2002.

20. Des Maisons, p. 62.

21. Blass, E. M., and A. Shah. "Pain-reducing properties of sucrose in human newborns," *Chemical Senses,* 20(1):29–35, 1995.

Blass, E. M., E. Fitzgerald, and P. Kehoe. "Interactions between sucrose, pain, and isolation distress" *Pharmacology, Biochemistry and Behavior,* 26:483–89. 1986.

22. "Formula in overweight and diabetes . . ." Bergmann, K. E., et al. "Early determinants of childhood overweight and adiposity in a birth cohort study: role of breast-feeding," *International Journal of Obesity and Related Metabolic Disorders,* 27(2):162–72, February 2003.

 Dietz, W. H. "Breastfeeding may help prevent childhood overweight," *Journal of the American Medical Association,* 285:2506–7, 2001.

 Von Kries, R., et al. "Breastfeeding and Childhood Obesity: A Systematic Review," *International Journal of Obesity,* 1–10, 2004.

23. Pettitt, D. J., and W. C. Knowler. "Long-term effects of the intrauterine environment, birth weight, and breast-feeding in Pima Indians," *Diabetes Care,* 21 Suppl 2:B138–41, August 1998.

24. Williams, Rebecca, and Isadora Stehlin. "Breast Milk or Formula: Making the Right Choice for Your Baby," Food and Drug Administration, fda.gov/fdac/reprints/breastfed .html, site accessed January 2006.

25. Ritter, J. L. "Critical Mass Traffic problems in the L.A. area can be alleviated by supporting public transportation projects," *UCLA Daily Bruin,* April 21, 1997.

26. In San Francisco, General Motors closed down the Key System public transit line. A history, "Traffic Engineers vs. Transit Patrons" can be found at trainweb.org/mts/ctc/ctc03 .html, site accessed January 2006.

 The same general process of the destruction of public transit happened throughout the US. A coalition of auto, gas, tire and highway construction companies created the modern car culture by force. Developers built new, transitless communities far from big cities. Then all these forces pushed through the massive highway construction projects of the 50s, 60s and 70s. The plot of the movie "Who Framed Roger Rabbit?" centered on this conspiracy.

27. "You can't walk; you are forced to drive." I recently visited some of these towns in Maryland and Ohio; children don't even walk two blocks to school — their parents drive them. See: Catlin, T.K., E.J. Simoes, and R.C. Brownson. "Environmental and policy factors associated with overweight among adults in Missouri," *Am J Health Promotion*, 17(4): 249–58, 2003.
28. Bell, A. C., K. Ge, and B. M. Popkin. "The road to obesity or the path to prevention: motorized transportation and obesity in China," *Obesity Research*, 10:277–283, 2002.

Chapter 4

1. Glasgow, R. E., E. Wagner, R. M. Kaplan, F. Vinicor, L. Smith, and J. Norman. "If diabetes is a public health problem, why not treat is as one? A population-based approach to chronic illness," *Annals of Behavioral Medicine*, 21:159–170, 1999.
2. Bernstein, Richard, M.D. *Dr. Bernstein's Diabetes Solution, Little*, Brown, 1997.
3. Payne, Craig, DPM. "Secrets To Fostering Self-Care In Patients With Diabetes," *Podiatry Today*, March 2001.
    Glasgow, Russell, and R. M. Anderson. "In diabetes care, moving from compliance to adherence is not enough," *Diabetes Care*, 22(12)2090–2091, 1999.
4. Aikens, James, Raymond Bingham, and John Piette. "Patient-Provider Communication and Self-Care Behavior Among Type 2 Diabetic Patients," *The Diabetes Educator*, 31 (5)681–690, September 2005.
5. Vermeire, E., P. Van Royen, S. Coenen, J. Wens, and J. Denekens. "The adherence of type 2 diabetes patients to their therapeutic regimens: a qualitative study from the patient's perspective," *Practical Diabetes International*, 20: 209–214, 2003.
6. Hiss, Roland, M.D. "The Concept of Diabetes Translation:

Addressing barriers to widespread adoption of new science into clinical care," *Diabetes Care,* 24:1293–1296, 2001.

7. Langer, Ellen. *The Psychology of Control,* SAGE Publications, 1983.

8. Steele, C. M., and J. Aronson. "Stereotype threat and the intellectual test performance of African Americans," *Journal of Personality and Social Psychology,* 69(5):797–811, November 1995.

9. Powell, M. Paige, S. Glover, J. Probst, and S. Laditka. "Barriers Associated with the Delivery of Medicare-Reimbursed Diabetes Self-Management Education," *The Diabetes Educator,* 31(6):890–899, November 2005.

10. Sanchez, C. D., et al. "Diabetes-related knowledge, atherosclerotic risk factor control, and outcomes in acute coronary syndromes," *Am J Cardiol,* 1;95(11):1290–4, Jun 2005.

11. Norris, S. L., M. M. Engelgau, and K. M. Narayan. "Effectiveness of self-management training in type 2 diabetes: a systematic review of randomized controlled trials," *Diabetes Care,* 24:561–587, 2001.

12. Three books on the subject of drug therapy dominance and corporate influence are:

Angell, Marcia, M.D. *The Truth About the Drug Companies: How They Deceive Us and What to Do About It,* Random House, 2004.

Abramson, John, M.D. *Overdosed America: the Broken Promise of American Medicine,* HarperCollins, 2005.

Critser, Greg. *Generation RX: How Prescription Drugs are Altering American Lives, Minds and Bodies,* Houghton Mifflin Company, 2005.

12A. Herman, W. H., et al., The Diabetes Prevention Group, "The cost-effectiveness of lifestyle modification or metformin in preventing type 2 diabetes in adults with impaired glucose tolerance," *Annals of Internal Medicine,* 142(5):323–32, March 1, 2005.

13. Bowman, Lee. "Most people with Type 2 diabetes fail to control blood sugar," *Scripps Howard News Service,* May 19, 2005.

14. The Diabetes Control and Complications Trial lasted ten years and generated hundreds of scientific papers. See: diabetes.niddk.nih.gov/dm/pubs/control, site accessed January 2006.

15. The UKPDS was an amazing study, lasting 20 years and generating dozens of valuable papers. See: dtu.ox.ac.uk/index.html?maindoc=/ukpds, site accessed January 2006.

16. Bodenheimr, Thomas, M.D. "High and Rising Health Care Costs. Part 1: Seeking an Explanation" *Annals of Internal Medicine,* 142(10):847–854 May 17, 2005.

17. Pollitz, Karen, Eliza Bangit, Kevin Lucia, Mila Kofman, Kelly Montgomery, and Holly Whelan. "Falling Through the Cracks: Stories of How Health Insurance Can Fail People with Diabetes," Georgetown University and American Diabetes Association, February 8, 2005. healthpolicywatch.org/research.asp?pubid=793, site accessed January 2006.

18. Urbina, Ian. "In the Treatment of Diabetes, Success Often Does Not Pay," *New York Times,* January 11, 2006.

19. Anderson, Gerard, Peter Hussey, Bianca Frogner, et al. "Health Spending in the United States and the Rest of the Industrialized World," *Health Affairs,* 24(4):903–14, July/August 2005.

20. Brown, Barry. "Canada's Way: What a universal health care system delivers, good and bad," *San Francisco Chronicle,* October 14, 2004.

21. For example, if you gave a drug to a group of 10,000 patients, and their blood pressures dropped by an average of eight points, it's very unlikely that this result happened by chance. There is perhaps less than a one in a thousand

chance of this occurring. (The exact chance would depend on statistical factors like the standard deviation, how variable the results were.) In this case, the p-value would be < .001, the results would be reported far and wide, and use of the drug would likely take off. Now, imagine a trial of 12 patients who are practicing meditation, and their blood pressures are lowered by an average of 15 points. Because there are only a few patients in the trial, these results could have happened by chance, perhaps as often as five percent of the time. The p-value would be 0.05, a much less impressive result than the larger study. The media and the medical profession would take no notice. Unlike the drug manufacturer in the earlier example, those advocating for meditation don't have a marketing department, so the positive outcome of their study would remain unknown.

22. See diabetes.org/nutrition-and-recipes/nutrition/starches.jsp, site accessed January 2006.

23. Some recent studies on intake of carbohydrates and fats and their effects on health factors are: Shah, M., et al. "Effect of a high-carbohydrate versus a high-*cis*-monounsaturated fat diet on blood pressure in patients with type 2 diabetes," *Diabetes Care*, 28(11):2607–12, November 2005.

24. Reaven, Gerald, et al. "Insulin resistance, dietary cholesterol, and cholesterol concentration in postmenopausal women," *Metabolism*, 50(5):594–7, May 2001.

25. Erlanson-Albertsson, C., and J. Mei. "The effect of low carbohydrate on energy metabolism," *International Journal of Obesity*, 29 Suppl 2:S26–30, September 2005.

26. Appel, L. J., et al. "Effects of protein, monounsaturated fat, and carbohydrate intake on blood pressure and serum lipids: results of the OmniHeart randomized trial," *Journal of the American Medical Association*, 294(19):2455–64, November 16, 2005.

27. Willett, Walter, and Meir Stampfer. "Rebuilding the Food

Pyramid: The dietary guide introduced a decade ago has led people astray. Some fats are healthy for the heart, and many carbohydrates clearly are not," *Scientific American,* December 17 2002.

28. Nestle, Marion. *Food Politics,* University of California Press, 2003.

29. Hu, F. B., R. M. van Dam, and S. Liu. "Diet and risk of Type II diabetes: the role of types of fat and carbohydrate," *Diabetologia,* 44(7)805–17, July 2001.

30. Mayers, Dara. "The nutrition advice given to most diabetics might be killing them," *U.S. News Health and Medicine,* July 14, 2003.

31. Dinsmoor, Robert. "Sulfonylureas," *Diabetes Self-Management,* September/October 1998.

32. Feinman, Richard, letter to *New York Times,* January 11, 2006. Mr. Feinman is a professor of biochemistry at SUNY Downstate Medical Center and co-editor of *Nutrition and Metabolism.*

32. McFarlane, S. I., et al. "Near-normoglycaemic remission in African-Americans with Type 2 diabetes mellitus is associated with recovery of beta cell function," *Diabetes Medicine,* 18(1):10–16 January 2001.

33. Anderson, Bob, and Martha Funnell. *The Art Of Empowerment: Stories And Strategies For Diabetes Educators,* American Diabetes Association, 2003.

Chapter 5

1. Puhl, R., and K. Brownell. "Bias, discrimination and obesity," *Obesity Research,* 9:788–805, 2001.

2. Anderson, R. J., K. E. Freedland, R. E. Clouse, and P. J. Lustman. "The prevalence of comorbid depression in adults with diabetes: a meta-analysis," *Diabetes Care,* 24(6):1069–78, June 2001.

3. Krein, S. L., M. Heisler, J. D. Piette, F. Makki, and E. A.

Kerr. "The effect of chronic pain on diabetes patients' self-management," *Diabetes Care,* 28(1):65–70, January 2005.

4. Blyth, F. M., L. M. March, A. J. Brnabic, L. R. Jorm, M. Williamson, and M. J. Cousins. "Chronic pain in Australia: a prevalence study," *Pain,* 89(2-3):127–34 January 2001.

5. Narayan, K. M., et al. "Randomized clinical trial of lifestyle interventions in Pima Indians: a pilot study," *Diabetes Medicine,* 15(1):66–72, January 1998.

6. *Creating Healthy Communities: An Alaskan Talking Circle,* Alaska Department of Health & Social Services, Division of Public Health, November 2002.

7. Smith, Barbara, Gloria Steinem, Gwendolyn Mink, Marysa Navarro, and Wilma Mankiller, eds. *The Reader's Companion to U.S. Women's History,* Houghton Mifflin Company 1998.
Ruiz, Vicki, and Ellen Dubois, eds. *Unequal Sisters: A Multicultural Reader in U.S. Women's History, 3rd Edition,* Routledge, February 2000.

8. Mori, Y, K. Hoshino, K. Yokota, T. Yokose, and N. Tajima. "Increased visceral fat and impaired glucose tolerance predict the increased risk of metabolic syndrome in Japanese middle-aged men," *Experimental and Clinical Endocrinology & Diabetes,* 113(6):334–9, June 2005.

9. Klein, S., L. Fontana, V. L. Young, A. R. Coggan, C. Kilo, B. W. Patterson, and B. S. Mohammed. "Absence of an effect of liposuction on insulin action and risk factors for coronary heart disease," *New England Journal of Medicine,* 17:350(25):2549–57, June 2004.

10. Gumbs, A.A., I.M. Modlin, and G.H. Ballantyne."Changes in insulin resistance following bariatric surgery: role of caloric restriction and weight loss," *Obesity Surgery,* 15(4): 462–73, April 2005.

11. Stevens, J., K. R. Evenson, O. Thomas, et al. "Association of fitness and fatness with mortality in Russian and American

men in the lipids research clinics study," *Int J Obes Relat Metab Disord* 28:1463–1470, 2004.

Blair, S. N., and S. Brodney. "Effects of physical inactivity and obesity on morbidity and mortality: current evidence and research issues," *Med Sci Sports Exerc*, 31 S646–62, 1999.

12. Gower, B. A., R. L. Weinsier, J. M. Jordan, G. R. Hunter, and R. Desmond. "Effects of weight loss on changes in insulin sensitivity and lipid concentrations in pre-menopausal African American and white women," *American Journal of Clinical Nutrition,* 76(5):923–7, November 2002.

13. "... the conventional model of beauty promotes a body that is far too thin..." Look back at pictures of the women who were considered sex symbols 50 or more years ago. All would be considered fat now. In cultures where food remains difficult to come by, fat is still considered attractive, at least in women, and most often in both sexes. Certainly, the current ideal contributes to eating disorders, which kill thousands of women every year in the US. Being underweight increases the statistical risk of death from many causes:

Flegal, K. M., B. I. Graubard, D. F. Williamson, M. H. Gail, "Excess deaths associated with underweight, overweight, and obesity," *Journal of the American Medical Association,* 293(15):1816–7, April 20, 2005.

14. Sikes, Ruth. *The History of Suntanning: A Love/Hate Affair,* skincarederm.com/history.htm, site accessed January 2006.

Chapter 6

1. "...90% of diabetes care is self-care..." This only an estimate. Some say 80%, other estimates are as low as 60%. But most everyone agrees that what people do for themselves is primary in diabetes. People are with themselves all the time; they only see doctors once in awhile.

2. "...self-confidence, a fundamental aspect of succeeding at self-care..." Most of the ideas in this chapter come from the following books and studies:

Bandura, Albert. *Self-Efficacy: The exercise of control,* W. H. Freeman, 1997.

Langer, Ellen. *The Psychology of Control,* SAGE Publishers, 1983.

Lorig, Kate, and Virginia Gonzalez. "The integration of theory with practice: a 12-year case study," *Health Education Quarterly,* 19(3):355–68, Fall 1992.

3. A thorough book on locus of control is: Lefcourt, Herbert. *Locus of Control: Current Trends in Theory and Research,* Lea, 1982.

4. "Stages of Change" is a current hot trend in behavioral change theory. It states that people who aren't ready to change, won't. So change agents should assess people's readiness to change and act appropriately (i.e., by not pushing change on those who aren't ready for it). Professors James O. Prochaska, Ph.D. of the University of Rhode Island and Carlo C. DiClemente, Ph.D. of the University of Maryland developed the theory and gave it the somewhat pretentious name "Transtheoretical Model." A Google or PubMed search for these terms or names will give hundreds of pages of information on the theory.

5. Bandura, Albert, R. W. Jeffery, and E. Gajdos. "Generalizing change through participant modeling with self-directed mastery," *Behav Res Ther,* 13(2-3):141–52, June 1975. In his book, *Self-Efficacy in Changing Societies,* Cambridge University Press 1997, the professor details how self-efficacy generalizes and why it often doesn't.

6. The Arthritis Self-Management Program started a revolution, of which this book is a part. The idea of using lay leaders instead of health professionals was particularly radical, and still has not been widely accepted by American medical

circles. See: Lorig, Kate, D. S Sobel, A. L. Stewart, B. W. Brown Jr., A. Bandura, P. Ritter, V. M. Gonzalez, D. D. Laurent, and H. R. Holman. "Evidence suggesting that a chronic disease self-management program can improve health status while reducing hospitalization: a randomized trial," *Med Care*, 37(1):5–14, January 1999.

7. "...vicarious accomplishment" and the use of lay leaders. See Bandura.

8. "SE practices work best when applied to behaviors..." ibid.

9. "...therapists or clergy members can help people reframe their stories..." See: Spero, David, RN. "How Stories Can Heal," *Diabetes Self-Management,* April-May 2004.

10. Maté, G. *When the Body Says No,* John Wiley & Sons, 2003. I owe Dr. Maté's book a lot for helping me to understand how early childhood experience sets people up for stress and disease in later life.

11. Polonsky, William, Ph.D. *Diabetes Burnout: Preventing It, Surviving It, Finding Inner Peace,* American Diabetes Association, 1999.

12. Langer, Ellen, and Judith Rodin. "Long-term effects of a control-relevant intervention with the institutionalized aged," *Journal of Personality and Social Psychology,* 37(11): 2003–13, November 1979.

13. Lynch, James, M.D. *A Cry Unheard: New Insights into the Medical Consequences of Loneliness,* Bancroft Press, 2000.

Chapter 7

1. Wolf, Stewart, and John Bruhn. *The Power of Clan: a 25-year prospective study of Roseto Pennsylvania,* Transaction Publishers, 1993.

2. The phrase "shelter of each other" comes from psychologist Mary Pipher's *The Shelter of Each Other: Rebuilding our families,* Random House, 1996.

3. Chesla, Catherine, L. Fisher, et al. "Family and disease

management in African-American patients with T2D," *Diabetes Care*, 27(2850–2855), December 2004.

Chesla Catherine, and K. M. Chun. "Accommodating Type 2 Diabetes in the Chinese American Family," *Quality Health Research*, 15(20)240–55, February 2005.

4. Rolnick, Art, and Rob Grunewald. "Early Childhood Development: Economic Development with a High Public Return," *fedgazette*, March 2003. minneapolisfed.org /pubs/fedgaz/03-03/earlychild.cfm, site accessed January 2006.

5. Wagner, Edward H., L. C. Grothaus, N. Sandhu, M. S. Galvin, M. McGregor, K. Artz, and E. A. Coleman. "Chronic care clinics for diabetes in primary care: a system-wide randomized trial," *Diabetes Care*, 24:695–700, 2001.

6. Trento, M., P. Passera, E. Borgo, M. Tomalino, M. Bajardi, F. Cavallo, and M. Porta. "A 5-year randomized controlled study of learning, problem solving ability, and quality of life modifications in people with type 2 diabetes managed by group care," *Diabetes Care*, 27(3):670–5, March 2004.

Trento, M., P. Passera, et al. "Lifestyle intervention by group care prevents deterioration of Type 2 diabetes: a 4-year randomized controlled clinical trial," *Diabetologia*, 45(9)1231–9, September 2002.

7. Clancy, Dawn E., D. W. Cope, K. M. Magruder, P. Huang, K. H. Salter, and A. W. Fields. "Evaluating group visits in an uninsured or inadequately insured patient population with uncontrolled type 2 diabetes," *Diabetes Educator*, 29(2):292–302, 2003 March-April.

8. Sadur, Craig N., N. Moline, M. Costa, D. Michalik, D. Mendlowitz, S. Roller, R. Watson, B. E. Swain, J. V. Selby, and W. C. Javorski. "Diabetes management in a health maintenance organization: efficacy of care management using cluster visits," *Diabetes Care*, 22:2011–2017, 1999.

9. Weinger, Katie, EdD, RN. "Group Medical Appointments in Diabetes Care: Is There a Future?" *Diabetes Spectrum,* 16:104–107, 2003.
10. Carlson, Bob. "Shared Appointments Improve Efficiency in the Clinic," *Managed Care,* May 2003.
11. Bell, Howard. "Group Appointments — Just What the Doctor Ordered," *Minnesota Medicine,* Vol. 85, June 2002.
12. Kilo, Charles, Dennis Horrigan, Marjorie Godfrey, and John Wasson. "Making Quality and Service Pay: Part 1, The Internal Environment," *Family Practice Management,* October 2000.
13. Martinez, Barbara. "Now It's Mass Medicine," *Wall Street Journal,* August 21, 2000.
14. Berwick, Donald. *Escape Fire: Designs for the Future of Health Care,* Jossey Bass, 2003.
15. *Arthritis Self-Help Course Leader's Manual and Reference Materials,* Arthritis Foundation, 1995.

Chapter 8

1. The *Amigos en Salud* results were presented at the Centers for Disease Control and Prevention Diabetes Translation Conference, May 5, 2005. See: pfizerhealthsolutions.com/main.htm, site accessed January 2006. Drug companies occasionally do some useful things, and I applaud them when they do. They certainly have the resources to do them.
2. walkingbus.com/links.htm, site accessed January 2006.
3. Webster, B. "Children on bicycles learn to beat the school-run blues," *The London Times,* June 17, 2002.
4. Lawless, Greg, and Anne Reynolds, "Keys to Successful Start-Ups for Rural Food Co-ops: Four Case Studies," Report CIR 63, University of Wisconsin Center for Cooperatives, rurdev.usda.gov/rbs/pub/sep05/taking.htm, site accessed January 2006.

Chapter 9

1. Chrstopher, MaryAnn, Judith Miller, and Theresa Beck. "Working with the Community for Change," in Mason, Diana, and Judith Leavitt, eds. *Policy and Politics in Nursing and Health Care, 3rd Edition*, Saunders, 1998.

2. "...a five-fold return on investment from their employee fitness program." — reported in *The Holland Sentinel,* Jul 13 2001. hollandsentinel.com/stories/071101/bus_071101003 5.shtml, registration required, site accessed January 2006.

3. Indy in Motion. See: indyfitness.net/home.htm, site accessed January 2006.

4. Colorado on the Move. See: americaonthemove.org/Affili ates.asp?AffiliateID=2, site accessed January 2006.

5. England cycling network. See: sustrans.org.uk/default.asp? sID=1090412763593, site accessed January 2006.

6. Robson, Judy Biros. "One Nurse's Journey to Becoming a Policymaker," in Mason, Diana, and Judith Leavitt, eds. *Policy and Politics in Nursing and Health Care, 3rd Edition,* Saunders, 1998.

7. Santora, Marc. "East Meets West, Adding Pounds and Peril," *New York Times,* January 12, 2006.

8. Fergusson, D. M., H. Grant, L. J. Horwood, and E. M. Ridder. "Randomized trial of the Early Start program of home visitation," *Pediatrics,* 116(6):803–9, December 2005.

9. Olds, D. L., et al. "Effects of nurse home-visiting on maternal life course and child development: age 6 follow-up results of a randomized trial," *Pediatrics,* 114(6):1550–9, December 2004.

10. nursefamilypartnership.org, site accessed January 2006.

11. Merrow, John. "European preschools should embarrass USA," *USA Today,* July 17, 2002.

12. *From Neurons to Neighborhoods: The Science of Early Childhood Development,* Institute of Medicine, 2002.

13. Kelder, Steven H. "History and Overview of CATCH: The

Coordinated Approach to Child Health," presentation at American Public Health Association 133rd Annual Meeting & Exposition, December 13, 2005.

14. Brownell, and Horgen, Chapter 5.

15. Farms to Schools. See: farmtoschool.org/index.htm, site accessed January 2006.

16. The National Family Farm Coalition. See: nffc.net/what/index.html, site accessed January 2006.

17. Penner, Tracy, and Ilene Pevec. "Gardens in Prison," City Farmer, Canada's Office of Urban Agriculture, cityfarmer.org/prison.html, site accessed January 2006

18. "Proceedings of the Roundtable on Understanding the Paradox of Hunger and Obesity," Food Research and Action Center, November 2005. frac.org/pdf/proceedings05.pdf, site accessed December 2005

19. Sebastian, Simone. "Boxing coach took charge of P.E., and an entire school changed," *San Francisco Chronicle,* January 25, 2006.

Chapter 10

1. *The Gift of Diabetes,* Brion Whitford, director, VHS 58 minutes, National Film Board of Canada, 2005. This is a really wonderful film.

2. Farley, S. S. "Leadership for Developing Citizen-Professional Partnerships: Perspective on Community," *Nursing and Health Care,* 16(4)226–228, June 1995.

Index

About the Author

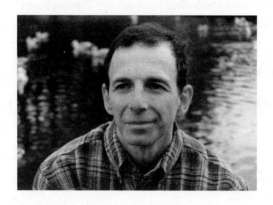

DAVID SPERO is a nurse living with multiple sclerosis; he knows chronic illness from inside and out. He is a community organizer, health care activist and journalist, writing regularly for *Diabetes Self-Management magazine*. His articles have also appeared in *Crossroads, Yes!, Alternative Medicine, RN,* the *San Francisco Bay Guardian,* and elsewhere.

Since the publication of his first book, *The Art of Getting Well: Maximizing Health When You Have a Chronic Illness* (Hunter House 2002), David has led self-management and wellness groups for patients and has trained health care providers in the US and Europe. He works with the Institute for Healthcare Improvement to help providers do a better job of helping patients help themselves. He is married with two grown children and lives in San Francisco.

If you have enjoyed *Diabetes: Sugar Coated Crisis*
you might also enjoy other

BOOKS TO BUILD A NEW SOCIETY

Our books provide positive solutions for people who want to
make a difference. We specialize in:

Environment and Justice • Conscientious Commerce
Sustainable Living • Ecological Design and Planning
Natural Building & Appropriate Technology • New Forestry
Educational and Parenting Resources • Nonviolence
Progressive Leadership • Resistance and Community

For a full list of NSP's titles, please call **1-800-567-6772** *or check out our website at:*

www.newsociety.com

NEW SOCIETY PUBLISHERS